# The Pandemic in Central Europe

This book studies the different models adopted by contemporary states in Central Europe in fighting the SARS-CoV-2 virus. With thorough analysis of different results and impacts of governmental policies, the authors examine the direction of the global economy after the pandemic ends.

The volume:

- Analyses the risks and effectiveness of the policy strategies taken by political regimes within the states of Central Europe;
- Probes into the changes in the functioning of post-pandemic society, especially the limitations of human rights due to state coercion and corruption risks;
- Understands issues related to the law-making process, healthcare policy, digitisation of state institutions and key processes carried out by entities of the system of public authority, and the establishment of principles and mechanisms of cooperation between the state and the business environment;
- Distinguishes the approaches of central and local administrations and of public authorities and citizens to the pandemic phenomenon;
- Assesses the actions taken by NATO and the national armed forces in the fight against the COVID-19 pandemic, with particular emphasis on the situation in the Visegrad Group countries.

A timely study, this will be of great interest to scholars and researchers of political theory, sociology, public health and social care, governance, public policy, security studies and public administration.

**Jolanta Itrich-Drabarek** is a Professor at the University of Warsaw. She is a political scientist and holds a PhD with "habilitation" in social science and is a Member of the Scientific Excellence Council of the 1st term.

# The Pandemic in Central Europe

Europe

A Case Study

Edited by Jolanta Itrich-Drabarek

Routledge
Taylor & Francis Group

LONDON AND NEW YORK

First published 2023
by Routledge
4 Park Square, Milton Park, Abingdon, Oxon OX14 4RN

and by Routledge
605 Third Avenue, New York, NY 10158

*Routledge is an imprint of the Taylor & Francis Group, an informa business*

*British Library Cataloguing-in-Publication Data*
A catalogue record for this book is available from the British Library

ISBN: 978-1-032-28768-3 (hbk)
ISBN: 978-1-032-40592-6 (pbk)
ISBN: 978-1-003-35381-2 (ebk)

DOI: 10.4324/9781003353812

Typeset in Sabon
by SPi Technologies India Pvt Ltd (Straive)

# Contents

Summary 192

JOLANTA ITRICH-DRABAREK

*Index* 194

# Illustrations

## Tables

## Charts

# List of contributors

**Marta Balcerek-Kosiarz** holds a post-doctoral degree in social science, is Assistant Professor at the Department of State Sciences and Public Administration at the Faculty of Political Science and International Studies, University of Warsaw.

**Jozefína Drotárová** holds a PhD, MBA and MPH and is Vice-rector for Science and Research (Department of Science and Research), University of Security Management in Košice (Slovakia).

**Jacek Dworzecki** is Professor of the Department of Public Administration and Crisis Management Academy of the Police Force in Bratislava.

**Paweł Hut** holds a post-doctoral degree in social science and is adjunct in Labour System and Labour Market Unit of Faculty of Political Sciences and International Studies, University of Warsaw, and is a political scientist and Member of the Refugee Board at Prime Minister Chancellary (2004–2019), Advisory Board in International Center of Migration Developement (2017–).

**Jolanta Itrich-Drabarek** is Professor and PhD with "habilitation" in social science, Vice-Dean for Development, Faculty of Political Sciences and International Studies, University of Warsaw, and a political scientist.

**Jacek Jastrzębski** holds a post-doctoral degree and is Professor in legal science at the Faculty of Law and Administration of the University of Warsaw. He also completed the Professional LLM law program at the University of California, Berkeley (2018). Since 2018, he serves as the Chairman of the Polish Financial Supervision Authority.

**Marcin Jurgilewicz** holds a post-doctoral degree in social sciences in the field of security science, and is Professor at the Rzeszów University of Technology, Dean of the Faculty of Management at the Rzeszów University of Technology (2019–2020) and Chairman of the Security Science Discipline Council of the Rzeszów University of Technology.

**Lucia Kurilovská** is Professor and JUDr., Rector of the Academy of the Police Force in Bratislava (since 2014) while also lecturing at the

Department of Penal Law of the Faculty of Law at Comenius University in Bratislava.

**Kamil Liberadzki** holds a post-doctoral degree and is Professor at the Warsaw School of Economics. He graduated from the Warsaw School of Economics (Finance and Banking Faculty) and the Law Faculty at the Warsaw University, Poland. He is a Member of the European Banking Authority (EBA) Board of Supervisors (BoS).

**Mojmír Mamojka** is Professor JUDr., Vice-rector for Science and Foreign Relations at the Academy of the Police Force in Bratislava while also lecturing at the Department of Business and Economic Law of the Faculty of Law at Comenius University in Bratislava.

**Ewa Maria Marciniak** holds a PhD with "habilitation" in social science in Faculty of Political Science and International Studies at Warsaw University, and is a political scientist specializing in the study of social communication and political behaviour and Former director of the Institute of Political Science at the University of Warsaw.

**Andrzej Misiuk** is Professor of humanities, Head of the Department of Security Science at the Institute of Political Science, University of Warsaw. Author of 60 compact works and over 200 scientific articles in the field of security, history and public administration.

**Kamil Mroczka** holds a PhD in political science and is Assistant Professor at the Faculty of Political Science and International Studies of the University of Warsaw, graduate of the Executive MBA programme offered by the International Management Center at the University of Warsaw and served as a Member of the Supervisory Board of Bank from 2017–2019.

**Justyna G. Otto** holds a PhD in humanities in the field of political science, is Assistant Professor at the Department of State Sciences and Public Administration at the Faculty of Political Sciences and International Studies, University of Warsaw, a political scientist, and also a journalist and an educator. In the years 2014–2021, Justyna served as Head of studies in Political Science and in the years 2015–2016 also as Head of the part-time 1st and 2nd degree studies in Internal Security.

**Marcin Tobiasz** holds a PhD in political sciences (2008), a research and teaching fellow at the Faculty of Political Science and International Studies of the University of Warsaw and in the years 2012–2016 served as Manager of undergraduate studies in Political Science and from 2016 to 2019, as Deputy Director of the Institute of Political Science.

# Introduction

*Jolanta Itrich-Drabarek*

This book is the first attempt to systematically define and explain the behaviour of political actors in different pandemic contexts, to identify similarities and differences between countries using Central Europe as an example, and to identify the sources and outcomes of these critical features. In its considerations, it focuses on the Visegrad Group countries. This territorial scope is supported by the uniqueness of this area manifested by the common experience of the specificity of the post-totalitarian state, a similar level of economic development and economic situation, as well as a high ethnic homogeneity of the countries in the region.

The authors of this study posed a number of research questions. What is driving the politicisation of the pandemic? Is there a link between the fight against SARS-CoV-2 and the ruling parties' policies on migrants, legal changes restricting human and civil rights but unrelated to the pandemic? Has the populism of those in power in the Visegrad countries reduced the effectiveness of the state in combating the pandemic? Do relatively young democracies succumb to greater temptation than other "old democracies" and restrict civil rights and freedoms to a much greater extent under the pretext of fighting the pandemic? What resources did the state have before the pandemic, what solutions to the crisis were provided for in the constitution and the legal system more broadly, what legitimacy did governments and the parliamentary majorities supporting them enjoy, how were radical or less radical moves motivated, how was government information incorporated into the existing communication system, etc.? How should one evaluate in retrospect the counteraction – in the Visegrad countries during the COVID-19 pandemic – of social problems such as migration, employment and unemployment, climate policy and the resolution of social problems (on the example of crime prevention, the situation of senior citizens, cultural-psychological problems)?

It was assumed that in addition to the problems associated with the pandemic caused by the SARS-CoV-2 coronavirus causing COVID-19 disease, which are universal in nature, many countries are characterised by a lack of coherent healthcare policies, increased susceptibility to breaking and circumventing existing laws, and a high degree of objectification of citizens because those in power perceive the dangers of a pandemic differently from

DOI: 10.4324/9781003353812-1

citizens and fail to harness the potential of society to fight it, governments unduly restrict freedom, human and civil rights, and the central government sees restrictions on contact with other countries and an increase in the power of the central executive at the expense of the judiciary, parliament and local government as an effective way to fight the pandemic. The management of restrictions in many states is chaotic, because those in power, who come from populist tendencies, make too little use of expert knowledge, are attached to an excessive belief in their own infallibility, and the measures they take are ad hoc.

It was assumed that the state faced many challenges in its contemporary history, which it did not have to face before, due to the acceleration of law-making processes and the increase in the number of errors resulting from this, on the one hand, and the return to the tradition of questioning official normativity on the other, as well as the change of priorities in health-care policy (the fight against COVID-19 – the collapse of treatment of other diseases), the acceleration of the digitalisation of the state and its institutions causing an increase in threats to information security, as well as a change of paradigms (principles) of cooperation between those in power and the business environment. The coronavirus pandemic also affected the processes and mechanisms of functioning of the state, public decision-making and public management, transferring them from a largely analogue world to the "digital world".

It was assumed that during the SARS-CoV-2 pandemic, there was a shift in the priorities of state social policy, as some social problems receded into the background (crime, chronic diseases, loneliness of the elderly, migration and climate change), while the cultural-psychological problems faced by a society under quarantine restrictions intensified. In times of pandemics, the cooperation of those in power with the media becomes crucial in order for the public to understand the impact of the pandemic and the government's policies to mitigate it. The role of the media in times of pandemics increases, as they can be an effective tool in the hands of those in power, thanks to which government decisions, such as the management of restrictions, vaccination, etc., become understandable to citizens, or the media can become an independent source of information controlling government policy. Each of such decisions, and all of them together, have, in the long run, implications for the social structure, income differentials between social groups and social categories, widening inequalities, the status of minority and disadvantaged groups. It is an impulse to rethink and to change the nature of the state, although not necessarily the projects subsequently implemented, as evidenced by the forecasts of reconstruction and reorganisation of the institutional order after 2008.

In the first chapter, "Central European countries in times of plague: a historical perspective", the author, Justyna G. Otto, attempts to assess the impact of major epidemics on the destiny of the state in world history. The aim of the chapter is to examine the universal features of pandemics in order to characterise, from a historical-political perspective, all those research problems dealt with in the subsequent chapters of the book on contemporary Central European countries in times of pandemics. In the presented chapter, the author subjects to a multifaceted analysis the role that epidemics and pandemics of infectious diseases have played in the life of the territories that today comprise the Central European states. This role is examined through the analysis of the most representative, in the author's opinion, cases of states which historically covered the territory of contemporary Central Europe. The author poses two fundamental research hypotheses. Firstly: the reaction of authorities during a pandemic did not change despite the passing of centuries and historical experience, because authorities are people and their nature does not change, they do not learn and do not want to learn from previous experiences, they do not store them in the collective and institutional memory, no conclusions are drawn from them and therefore the outbreak of a pandemic comes as a surprise; the authorities still make decisions with a delay in relation to the development of events. Secondly, during a pandemic, the most appropriate and effective actions are those that take place at the lowest level of state organisation, locally, as close as possible to the people affected in a particular place, because this is what centuries of experience of fighting epidemics of plague, cholera, typhus, influenza and smallpox, experienced by the countries of Central Europe, teach us.

The second chapter, "Countries in Central Europe and the pandemic", by Marta Balcerek-Kosiarz, analyses the role of selected countries in Central Europe during the pandemic. On the example of Poland, the Czech Republic, Slovakia and Hungary (the Visegrad Group), the problem of legitimising governmental actions is presented, the analysis of governmental strategies to combat the pandemic is made, and irregularities and abuses of power which resulted from their implementation are pointed out.

In the third chapter, "Management of restrictions during the SARS-CoV-2 pandemic in Central European countries", the authors, Andrzej Misiuk, Marcin Jurgilewicz and Jozefína Drotárová, point to the need for an all-society discussion on changing the current security and health strategies and reconfiguring security systems. They assume that a responsible health and security policy cannot consist only in limiting the rights and freedoms of individuals, isolating the infected and quarantining those suspected of being infected, spending billions of dollars on unreliable vaccines and ad hoc anti-crisis measures aimed only at protecting systems critical to the security and functioning of the state from a severe overload. They emphasise that epidemiological protection legislation in Central European countries opens up a wide field of action for those in power, while the underdevelopment of alternative, so-called post-normal research infrastructures means that the study base available to decision-makers is limited, so that they lack high-quality scientific information about the effectiveness of available ways of limiting transmission and spread of the virus in the population, and about the legal, social, economic and political consequences of their choice and introduction. They discuss the ways in which the management of restrictions during the pandemic is legitimised, the intensity of the use of physical political violence and the measures used by state actors to prevent a pandemic. They attempt to discuss the legitimacy of restrictions on freedoms, human and civil rights during a pandemic, in relation to their abuse for political purposes, including the use of the pandemic for surveillance of citizens, the perception of threats by policy makers, and an analysis of state attitudes towards "outsiders".

The aim of the fourth chapter, "Major challenges facing states in pandemic conditions", authored by Jacek Jastrzębski, Kamil Mroczka, Kamil Liberadzki, is to examine and discuss issues related to the law-making process, healthcare policy, digitisation of state institutions and key processes carried out by the entities of the system of public authority, and to establish the principles and mechanisms of cooperation between the state and the business environment. The authors assumed that *the modern state, in relation to the pandemic of the coronavirus SARS-CoV-2 causing COVID-19 disease, faced the greatest challenges in its modern history, which it did not have to face before, because, on the one hand, there was an acceleration of law-making processes and an increase in the number of errors resulting from this, on the other hand, a return to the tradition of questioning official normativity, a change in healthcare policy priorities (the fight against COVID-19 – a collapse in the treatment of other diseases), an acceleration of the digitalisation of the state and its institutions resulting in an increase in threats to information security, and a change in paradigms (principles) of cooperation between those in power and the business environment. The coronavirus pandemic has also affected the processes and mechanisms of functioning of the state, public decision-making and public management, moving them in large part from the analogue world to the "digital world".*

In chapter five, entitled "Solving social problems during a pandemic", Paweł Hut hypothesised that the COVID-19 pandemic triggered profound changes in the perception of social problems. Decision-makers responsible for the field of social policy made significant re-evaluations in the implementation of previous tasks. Social problems – such as migration or climate protection, labour market protection, as well as cultural and social problems resulting from the reorganisation of social life and the imposed social isolation – became one of the greatest challenges. It is important, from the author's point of view, to assess the course and similarities and differences in the activities of the authorities of individual states. Reactivity and spontaneity, as well as individual and particular counteracting of the pandemic on the territory of individual states, should be regarded as a common element of the activities of V4 countries.

Chapter 6, "State and society in times of a pandemic", by Ewa Maria Marciniak and Marcin Tobiasz, assumes that the course of the pandemic in Poland, the Czech Republic, Slovakia and Hungary was similar, while the countermeasures differed. Among the similarities in the fight against the pandemic in the V4 countries one can point out closure of borders, restrictions on transport and movement of the population, the timely suspension of businesses in the tourism and gastronomy industries and the introduction of lockdown, a ban on cultural and sporting meetings and events, as well as the implementation of remote classes in secondary and higher education or hybrid lessons in primary education. The differences that have occurred in the fight against the pandemic in the countries of Central and Eastern Europe correspond to countermeasures such as carrying out universal diagnostics (the Czech Republic, Slovakia), vaccination campaigns (Poland, the Czech Republic, Slovakia, Hungary) and introduction of a state of emergency (the Czech Republic, Slovakia). The impact of the pandemic has deeper consequences in those countries where, prior to the pandemic, there was an inadequate level of health care, shortage of medical staff and lack of medical equipment. All the internal problems of the countries, which existed before the coronavirus, were highlighted and emphasised during the pandemic and became the main focus of the fight against the pandemic – i.e. by improving the situation internally, an attempt was made to solve the external problem, which was the SARS-CoV-2 virus.

The last – seventh – chapter, "The situation and role of the armed forces during the pandemic", by an international team of researchers Jacek Dworzecki, Mojmír Mamojka and Lucia Kurilovská, attempts to assess the actions taken by NATO and individual armed forces of the Visegrad Group in the fight against the COVID-19 pandemic in 2020. The analysis was based on the available literature on the subject, legal acts, media reports and several expert interviews with soldiers and civilian personnel of the armed forces from Poland and Slovakia as well as other persons working or serving in uniformed formations who cooperated with soldiers in pandemic-related activities.

The book reveals the results and indicates directions for future research on the role of the state in Central Europe. The authors of individual chapters point to the specificity of the countries of Central and Eastern Europe, define its sources and analyse the risks associated with the management of restrictions during a pandemic. They point to the role of the state in combating pandemics, make an attempt to explain the problems faced by political power and society and point to the dangers of abusing power during an emergency situation such as a pandemic. The fourth wave of the pandemic shows that the lessons of the first three have not been learnt, the governments of Central Europe are still not pursuing a consistent policy towards its manifestations and the pandemic of the unvaccinated has dominated its course.

# 1 Central European countries in times of plague

## A historical perspective

*Justyna G. Otto*

As Hans Zinsser wrote:

> (...) Swords and lances, bows and machine guns, even explosives had less effect on the fate of nations than the typhus louse, the plague flea and the yellow fever mosquito. Civilisation was retreating from the creeping disease of cholera, and armies were falling to pieces, becoming a disorderly fat lot before the attack of the cholera comma or the germ of dysentery or typhoid.
>
> (Michalski, 2009)

In the past, epidemics and pandemics did not spare the territories which today are occupied by countries such as Poland, Slovakia, the Czech Republic and Hungary, i.e. Central Europe. They affected not only the history of this region, shaping it, but also the functioning of states, their institutions, the lives of people, entire societies and local communities. Throughout human history epidemics and pandemics have fundamentally determined the fate of societies, families and individuals also in Central Europe.

The aim of this chapter is to examine the universal features of pandemics in order to characterise, from a historical and political perspective, all those research problems dealt with in the subsequent chapters of the book on contemporary Central European countries in times of a pandemic.

In this chapter, the author conducts a multifaceted analysis of the role that epidemics and pandemics of infectious diseases have played in the life of the territories that today comprise Central European states. This role is examined through the analysis of the most representative, in the author's opinion, cases of states which historically covered the territory of contemporary Central Europe. The borders of the states changed, shifted – there were partitions, invasions, etc. – but the tendencies remained the same.

In the following subsections, the author asks auxiliary research questions: What epidemics of infectious diseases, and when, did the states of Central Europe experience throughout history? How did these experiences place Central Europe and its constituent states in comparison with the world and, above all, with the rest of the Old Continent? Where did the inhabitants of

DOI: 10.4324/9781003353812-2

Central Europe see the causes of infectious diseases? What were they for them? How did individual citizens, families, smaller and larger communities, whole societies, as well as state and local authorities, secular and clerical elites, behave in the face of epidemics and pandemics? How did they react from the perspective of the individual, the group, cities, states? The detailed research questions are intended to lead the author to answer the central research questions of the chapter: Did Central Europe learn anything from the experiences of epidemics and pandemics that it faced in the past? How much, and whether at all, do the experiences of pandemics in the 21st century and those in earlier centuries differ in essence? In fact, does the immutability of human nature cause us to find in the experiences of Central Europe from centuries past a mirror image of the contemporary fight against the pandemic caused by the COVID-19 virus?

The author poses two main research hypotheses. Firstly, the reaction of authorities during a pandemic did not change despite the passing of centuries and historical experience, because authorities are people and their nature does not change, they do not learn and do not want to learn from previous experiences, they are not stored in the collective and institutional memory, no conclusions are drawn from them and therefore the outbreak of the pandemic takes them by surprise; the authorities still make decisions which do not keep up with the development of events. Secondly, during a pandemic, the most appropriate and effective actions are those taking place at the lowest level of state organisation, locally, as close as possible to the people affected in a particular area, because this is what the centuries of experience of fighting the plague, cholera, typhus, influenza and smallpox epidemics in the countries of Central Europe teach us.

## 1.1 The world, Europe and Central Europe: Epidemics of infectious diseases as an experience of Central Europe

From a historical perspective, Central Europe was mainly affected by epidemics of the plague, cholera, typhus, influenza and smallpox. And so, the plague has accompanied man since time immemorial. The DNA of the bacilli of this disease was discovered in the remains of a woman from around 5,000 years ago. Since ancient times, dozens of major epidemics known as the "black death" have been described, although we are not always sure whether it was the plague. By far the most tragic in its consequences was the great plague epidemic of 1348–1352, which covered the entire Mediterranean basin. According to the famous Polish medical historian and physician Władysław Szumowski (1875–1954), it was "the most terrible plague ever known to mankind". It reached Poland in 1349 (Nawrocka, 2008).

Exceptionally in Poland, that epidemic is believed to have passed almost unnoticed. This is attributed to the quarantine ordered by King Casimir the Great. For centuries, Poles have been fond of talking about Casimir the Great as an exceptional ruler, knowledgeable about medicine and epidemics, and prudently protecting his people from the plague. According to Katarzyna Pękacka-Falkowska from the Department of History and Philosophy of Medical Sciences at the Poznań University of Medical Sciences, nothing confirms the emerging hypotheses about globally unique methods of fighting the plague pandemic on the Polish soil.

> Most likely there were no quarantines, sanitary cordons or health passports for people and transported goods. Technically, on a large scale, such measures were not possible until the 17th century. I do not think that the king could have introduced any preventive measures on a supra-local scale. This would require resources that were not available at the time: a well-tailored administrative apparatus, services using direct coercion, the rapid circulation of information, and so on. In medieval Poland, the only preventive measures were flight and voluntary isolation.
>
> (Szczęsny, 2020)

A lot of information about serious epidemics in the second half of the 14th and the first half of the 15th centuries can be found in *Roczniki czyli kroniki sławnego Królestwa Polskiego* (Annals, or Chronicles of the Famous Kingdom of Poland) by Jan Długosz.[1] An entry for 1360 reads:

> Mór straszny w Polsce (…) zaraza (…) rozgościła się w Polsce, Węgrzech, Czechach, tudzież podległych im i sąsiedzkich ziemiach (…) Tem zaś różniła się ta klęska od poprzedniej, która przed laty dwunastą kraj nasz nawiedziła, że tamta wiele sprzątnęła ludzi z pospolitego gminu, od tej zaś więcej szlachty i ludzi możnych, dzieci i kobiet wyginęło. (A terrible plague in Poland (…) the plague (…) took root in Poland, Hungary, Bohemia, as well as neighbouring lands subordinate to them (…) What made this calamity different from the previous one which struck our country twelve years ago is that the former cleaned out many people from the common folk, while this one brought the death of more noblemen and wealthy people, children and women".)
>
> (Rosalak, 2020)

Historical sources record the occurrence of epidemics in Central Europe practically several to a dozen times in each century. The pestilence was particularly intense in the 16th and 17th centuries, when every few years there would be a plague of smaller, local or larger, nationwide scope. In Krakow, for example, 92 epidemics were recorded between 1500 and 1750. Historians estimate that in the 14th and 15th centuries, the then Polish lands were free from epidemics for 70 out of 100 days, and in the following two centuries for about 50 out of 100 days. There were centuries when the plague[2] appeared even 20 times, sometimes lasting even 2–3 years.

The plague attacked Europe a few times in the 15th century and a dozen or so times in the 16th and 17th centuries. Its worldwide apogee was between 1501 and 1650.[3] With this last epidemic, the plague withdrew from Western Europe but continued to take its deadly toll in the East. It took its toll, of course, during the Thirty Years' War (Nawrocka, 2008). In 1701, it attacked Constantinople; in 1703–1704, it raged in Ukraine; then it spread to Poland (1706) (Górski, 2008; Pękacka-Falkowska, 2019; Popiołek, 2016), Bohemia, Hungary, Austria (in Central Europe, Austria was affected at the latest in 1716 (Ruffié & Sournia, 1996) and Prussia. It also ravaged Ukraine, Hungary, Moravia, Austria and Poland from 1738 to 1744 (Naphy & Spicer, 2004). The last epidemic to affect Polish lands took place in Volhynia and Podolia between 1770 and 1771. By the end of the 18th century, the plague still appeared in the Balkans, Turkey and southern Russia but did not have the symptoms of a pandemic.

The disease was spread by the migratory black rat. It was probably its extinction at the end of the 18th century that brought the plague epidemics worldwide to a halt. The plague is transmitted to humans from rats via fleas, but it was not until the late 19th century that humans gained this knowledge. According to some researchers, the characteristic cyclical occurrence of the plague, every 10–15 years, was the result of the length of time a recovered person gained immunity to a new infection. Indeed, surviving the disease gave 10–15 years of immunity (Ruffié & Sournia, 1996). The plague usually appeared in spring or summer and lasted 4–7 months, as the frost destroyed the bacteria. The pneumonic plague, on the other hand, claimed most victims in winter, as did smallpox, typhus and influenza. The plague epidemics in Europe died out by the early 19th century. By then the Black Death had taken a terrible toll.[4] The plague was to return to Europe in the following decades but on an incomparably smaller scale. Cholera epidemics were to become the nightmare of the 19th century.

At the beginning of the 1820s, accounts of merchants travelling to India and South-East Asia describe a disease that manifested as vomiting, diarrhoea, weight loss and spots on the body. Arab sailors called it *kholera*, which means "leakage of bile" (Ruffié & Sournia, 1996). Its expansion began from the farthest regions of Asia, including Japan, which was closed to the world. It was one of the fastest spreading and most dangerous pathogens in the world (Colwell, 1996). In 1830, it reached Russia and later the rest of Europe. The exotic disease was initially treated as a harmless curiosity from the farthest end of the world. The wealthy bourgeoisie of Europe at that time thought that cholera took its toll only among the lowest circles of society. However, Prince Konstantin Romanov, who had fled Warsaw in November 1830 and observed the Russian army's actions against the November insurgents, died of the disease already in 1831. At almost the same time, on 10 June 1831, Field Marshal Ivan Dybicz Zabalkanski, commanding the tsarist army, died. Also in 1831, cholera took the lives of great representatives of Prussian intellectual life – Carl von Clausewitz and Georg Wilhelm Hegel (Zwoliński, 2020). The greatest Polish bard, Adam Mickiewicz, who died in Istanbul in 1855, was probably a victim of one of the subsequent waves of the plague. As Sonia Shah writes: "in 1830 Russian soldiers marched into Poland (to suppress the Polish independence uprising – comment by J.G. Otto). Cholera followed them like a spectre" (Faron, 2021; Shah, 2020; Wnęk, 2015).

Cholera was much more often fatal in the cities than in the countryside, which was the reason for the mass movement of the population, as with the plague. These changes in social structure and ethnic and linguistic balance did not always take place peacefully. When considering the history of Central Europe, it is worth mentioning the example of Austria-Hungary, where, in a mosaic of nations, German became the language of the administration and the elite. Here, in 1831, cholera killed some 250,000 people, mostly in the cities. In Hungary, the place of the dead was taken by peasants who came to the cities and spoke Hungarian. The same thing happened in Bohemia to Slavic languages. W.H. McNeill put forward a thesis that in the middle of the 19th century, a completely new distribution of nationalities took place in Central Europe and the Balkans in the course of one generation, and that cholera was therefore the cause of the break-up of the Viennese monarchy (Ruffié & Sournia, 1996).

Cholera pandemics represented a breakthrough in thinking about the prevention of infectious diseases. In 1854, the British physician John Snow began investigating the spread of cholera in the poorest districts of London. In his opinion, the theory of miasmas, or the causation of disease by "bad air", which had been functioning since the Middle Ages, was wrong. He succeeded in identifying the source of the plague – a well located at the epicentre of infections (Shah, 2020). Over the next few decades, the discovery of the causes of cholera led to the start of the fight against the epidemic by, among other things, building modern waterworks and sewage systems. City planners and architects also strove to make buildings more sparse, for example, by building parks. In cities, regulations were also introduced that prohibited pouring waste into gutters or directly into the street. In the largest centres, and later in smaller towns in Central Europe, the quality of water and food began to be controlled. More and more activities were undertaken by state institutions, for example, issuing sanitary regulations in case of an epidemic. For example, regulations that were in force in Lviv in 1910 stated that anyone suspected of having cholera should be reported to the county political authority.

During the first cholera epidemic in Poland in 1831–1838 (compare Olkowski, 1968) in the Kingdom of Poland alone about 13,000 people out of 4 million inhabitants died, but in Galicia more than 100,000 died out of the same number of inhabitants. The second epidemic in 1847–1849 (Faron, 2021) occurred during a famine. It is difficult to estimate the number of victims, as people also died from hunger and a simultaneous typhus epidemic. There were probably more dead victims than during the first epidemic. The third cholera pandemic in 1852–1860 may have claimed up to 200 million lives. This is considered the deadliest outbreak of infections in the world. It started in India, from where it moved to Russia and then to

Europe. Successive cholera epidemics on the Polish territory took place in 1866 and 1873, claiming tens of thousands of victims in Galicia alone. The last epidemic of 1892–1894 was small in Poland, but in Russia, for example, it killed 250,000 infected people.

In the 19th century, pestilence continued to pose a huge threat to social order. In 1846, a cholera epidemic struck Małopolska and Podhale. It was preceded by disastrous crop failures and floods. In many places, hunger riots broke out, which eventually turned into the Galician slaughter. The chaos was compounded by population migrations, which carried the germs to other areas.

Overall, cholera killed around 40 million people in Europe in the 19th century. Statistically, every 30th Pole died during a cholera epidemic in Poland. At the beginning of the 20th century, cholera disappeared in Europe, retreating to Asia, mainly to India.

As far as typhus is concerned, this disease, also known as spotted fever, is unknown to most people today, but in past eras it had a clear impact on the fate of empires from Napoleon to Lenin. The disease is transmitted by lice, and as we know, people and lice have long lived in close relationships (Allen, 2016). Typhus can be counted among the deadliest diseases in the history of mankind. Up to 50% of those infected died among the poorest populations. Although it was recognised only in the 20th century, and isolated as a separate disease in the 19th century, it has been taking a deadly toll, mainly among the poor and during wars, since antiquity (Treder, 2012). The chroniclers of the time referred to it as "camp fever", "ship fever" or "prison fever".[5] During the Great War, it decimated the population and soldiers on the Eastern Front in particular (Rosalak, 2020). Already in 1914, about 200,000 Serbian soldiers and Austrian prisoners of war died. In the following years, about 10 million people died of typhus in war-torn and revolutionary Russia.[6] During the First World War, despite the already known way in which the bacteria spread and doctors' recommendations, typhus appeared in the ranks of all fighting armies, killing the most soldiers in the Russian army: 2.5–3 million.

In the 19th century, two great typhus epidemics swept through Poland: in 1830–1831 and 1842–1846. The year 1916 brought another wave of the disease, with more than 26,000 typhus cases reported in Warsaw alone. At the same time, more than 34,000 patients were reported in Galicia and the Congress Poland. A year later, the number doubled, and when Poland regained independence, the epidemic raged for good. In 1918, there were 230,000 cases, of which nearly 20,000 ended in death. In 1919, 431,000 cases were registered, including 19,000 deaths (Berner, 2008). Most people fell ill in the Eastern Borderlands and in Lesser Poland, which was directly related to the reparation of prisoners of war and the return of many refugees from the East. Compared to Poland, only Russia had a higher incidence. In 1920, it was brought to Poland by Tuchaczewski's troops. During the Polish-Bolshevik War (1920), more people died from typhus than from the warfare.

As far as the influenza virus is concerned, it too has accompanied mankind for centuries, bringing suffering and death to millions of lives. The first records of influenza can be found as early as in the 5th century BC by Hippocrates, who in his work *Corpus Hippocraticum* introduced the term "Perinthos cough" to describe an upper respiratory tract infection (see Adams, 1886). Most European countries were haunted by periodic influenza epidemics. Among the more important ones, a large influenza pandemic occurred in Russia in the years 1729–1730. It was characterised by a secondary wave of infections, which occurred after two years and affected most European countries. The disease reached Poland in November 1732. In 1733 the pandemic reached America and Africa.

The largest influenza invasion in the 18th century is considered to be the pandemic of 1781–1782. The disease was called "instant catarrh": in autumn the first cases were reported in India, in December already in Russia, in January 1782 in St. Petersburg, in February in Finland, then the wave of the epidemic passed through Poland, Denmark, Germany, Sweden, England, Austria, the Netherlands, France, Spain and finally Italy. The scale of infections was enormous, and in many cities almost the entire population was ill. Along with the countless advantages of the development of civilisation, there were also disadvantages. A key factor in the subsequent spread of influenza was the development of transport and the consequent ease of travel. Thus, in the 19th century, the spread of the disease was even greater. The first pandemic took place between 1830 and 1833, starting in China (Brydak, 2008), then passing through, among others, the Philippines, India and Indonesia, reaching Europe via Russia and, as before, also affecting North America. Although the fatality rate was not exceptionally high this time, the morbidity rate was impressive, hovering around 20–25%.

At the end of the 19th century, the so-called Russian flu broke out. The epidemic also raged in Polish cities. At the beginning of December 1889, it appeared in Łódź and Warsaw, and then in Krakow and Poznań. In the capital city of Greater Poland, the epidemic reached its peak in mid-January but slowly subsided and was almost extinct by the end of the month. The disease was caused by a mutated H2 virus, unlike the H1 virus, which had previously been the culprit in seasonal influenza. Between 1889 and 1890, the number of fatalities exceeded 1,000,000.

The great movements of mass populations also contributed to the rapid expansion of the most terrible pandemic of the last 200 years, namely the Spanish flu in the years 1918–1919 (Shah, 2020). It was the largest influenza epidemic in modern times, and Spain, neutral in the Great War, was the only country that did not censor press coverage of infections, which is why the public initially believed this country to be the source of the disease. Spain reported on the spread of the epidemic (Brown, 2019; Wright, 2020). Its spread was facilitated precisely by the fact that the countries involved in the armed conflict did not make public reports on the extent of the epidemic and thus did not cooperate in combating it. The epidemic claimed around 50–100 million victims (Aberth, 2012; Brydak, 2008; Mieszkowski, 2020), which is more than the number of deaths during the First World War, while around 500 million people, or 25% of the then population, were infected. It was caused by the H1N1 avian influenza virus, which mutated and spread to humans. The flu was spread by troops returning from the frontlines after the end of hostilities. People died mainly from complications, especially from pneumonia. The highest mortality rate, as in any epidemic, was in large communities, which at the time included military camps, where sanitary conditions were also terrible. After the end of the war, soldiers returning home spread the virus throughout Europe and further around the world.

Therefore, most probably, contrary to what the name would suggest (Collier, 1974), the virus was brought to the Old Continent from the USA by American soldiers (Jasiński, 2019). The Spanish flu was different from the majority of pandemics in the history of the world, because its victims were not the weakest and burdened with serious diseases, but, above all, young and middle-aged people, in the age group of 20–40 years (Aberth, 2012; Wnęk, 2014). One of the hypotheses explaining this phenomenon is that older people had immunity to the Spanish flu acquired during the epidemic of the so-called Russian flu. The ease with which the virus was transmitted led to a situation where approximately one-third of the then Earth's population fell ill with this extremely dangerous type of flu. The death rate was increased by the fact that the Spanish flu fell on European societies weakened by terrible living conditions during the First World War. There was a shortage of food and medicines.

Today, it is virtually impossible to establish the number of victims of the Spanish flu in Central Europe, which is undoubtedly due, among other things, to the chaos of the first months of Poland's independence, the great migrations and other changes in the political map of Central Europe after the end of the First World War – the collapse of the great powers, the emergence of new independent states, and then the sweeping frontline of the war with the Bolsheviks – these events obliterated most of the traces of the plague. In addition, during the Second World War, most documents were destroyed (Mieszkowski, 2020), for example, those of the largest cemeteries in Warsaw, which would have provided an excellent source for estimating the mortality rate of the inhabitants of the Polish capital. The Spanish flu epidemic is therefore known to us almost only from memoirs and the press of the time. For example, the Krakow's *Głos Narodu* (Voice of the Nation) reported in its evening edition of 22 October 1918 that there was not a single household in the Sokal district near Lviv in which someone wouldn't have fallen with the Spanish flu. Usually, all the inhabitants of a given hut succumbed to it one by one. The mortality rate was enormous. Whole communities lay in high fever, many sufferers had blood coming out of their mouths and noses. The disease emaciated the population to such an extent that they were unable to work for a long time and the farm economy suffered. Potatoes were not dug, they rotted, and no crops were planted for the winter crops. The press reported that funerals were usually held without weeping, as often the whole family of the deceased lay in fever and there was no one to weep over the coffin. It was not uncommon for a mother lying unconscious in a fever not to know that her dead child was being carried out of the house. Whole families were ill in towns and villages, which affected every social group. Carpenters in villages and towns made nothing but coffins. The population succumbed to a feeling of complete apathy as there was no way to prevent the pestilence. Obituaries of a husband and wife or two or three children were published in the newspapers. Often death came very quickly. "In the morning you are healthy, in the evening you are gone" (Wnęk, 2014) – it was said at the time.

Many tried to use the epidemic to advertise secretly produced medical preparations and even their restaurants. One of Krakow's establishments advertised in the *Ilustrowany Kurier Codzienny* (Daily Courier Illustrated) that "hygienic and tasty" dishes protected against the disease.[7] Fear was also quenched with humour: "Przyszła kryska na Matyska: hiszpanka za szyję ściska/Ja się nie dam – krzyczał z pychą/Aż i jego wzięło licho" ("The pitcher may go once too often to the well: Spanish flu is clutching at his neck/I won't give in – he shouted with pride/Until he too was taken by the devil"), reads a poem in the *Kurier Poznański* (Poznan's Courier).[8]

The memory of the Spanish flu is present in Warsaw folklore: "My, warszawiacy, jesteśmy tacy/Kto nam na odcisk – to już Hiszpan – zimny trup" [Mieszkowski, 2020] ("We, the Varsovians, are like that/Whoever gets on the wrong side of us – is already a Spaniard – a cold corpse") – to this day, bands inspired by the music of the capital's backyards sing. Poems composed during previous epidemics of influenza were also recalled. "O influenzo, Nimfo, skąd Ty rodem? Czyś Ty chorobą jest epidemiczną? Co Ci się stało? Co Ci jest powodem? /Że tak w grodzie samym, jako też i w okolicy, marnujesz mężów, dzieci i kobiety?" ("O influenza, Nymph, where do you come from? Are you an epidemic disease? What has happened to you? What is the reason?/That in the castle-town itself, as well as in the neighbourhood, you waste husbands, children and women?") – wrote an anonymous author, paraphrasing a fragment of Juliusz Słowacki's *Beniowski*. The content of the poem makes us realise that it was not until the end of the 19th century that the mechanisms of transmission of the common flu were known. Before that, it was one of the many mysteries of medicine.

Historians assume that in 1918–1920, around 2,000 people died from Spanish flu in Warsaw, which had a population of over 820,000 at the time.

The Polish press alarmed: "Whole communes lie in enormous fever, many sick people gush blood from their mouths and noses. Anyone who catches a cold is going to the next world" (Wnęk, 2014). Influenza reached Lviv in the summer of 1918, Krakow in September and Warsaw in October. The wave of illnesses lasted until January 1919. Today, it is estimated that Spanish flu killed around 500,000 Poles (compare Mieszkowski, 2020).

The epidemic of 100 years ago has been exploited politically to this day. During the Polish-Bolshevik War, losses due to the pestilence among Bolshevik prisoners of war in Poland amounted to around 16,000–18,000 out of a total of 85,000. On the territory of Russia and Lithuania, almost 51,000 Polish soldiers were held in prisoner-of-war camps during this period, and up to 20,000 of them died as a result of the disease. For contemporary Russia, the enormous losses of Soviet soldiers are a pretext for putting forward theories about those prisoners having been allegedly starved to death by Poles. This thesis is an element of the Russian "anti-Katyn" narrative – the alleged murders committed on the orders of the Polish authorities 20 years before the crime against the Polish POWs (Zwoliński, 2020).

The only way to combat the epidemic was the introduction of extremely strict isolation rules, which were, however, difficult to enforce in very densely populated cities. The pandemic disappeared at the end of 1920 and never returned in similar intensity. In the following decades, however, dangerous influenza epidemics reached Poland again. The two most severe (H2N2 and H3N2), in 1957 and 1969, came from Asia. The latter claimed about 1,300 lives in Poland.

Smallpox was also a cause of concern for ancient societies. It was the cause of about 15% of deaths in European populations. The mortality rate reached 30%.[9] At the beginning of the 17th century, the so-called variolation began to gain popularity. The procedure consisted in implanting smallpox pustule fluid under the skin. The person subjected to such a vaccination underwent a mild variant of smallpox and gained permanent immunity (Aberth, 2012). The procedure was so popular that it was even used by the rulers of the time, such as the Russian Empress Catherine II. At the end of the 1760s, it was also carried out by the doctor of the Polish King Stanisław August Poniatowski (Gambal-Różańska, 2008). However, the procedure was quite risky. The mortality rate of "mild" smallpox was about 3%, which today may seem a shockingly high percentage but was almost negligible for people who lived in societies of huge epidemic risk.

Edward Jenner's improvement of vaccination (see: Aberth, 2012; Ruffié & Sournia, 1996) at the end of the 18th century began the process of global fight against smallpox, which ended with its defeat in 1978. This moment was predicted by Jenner himself when he claimed that the end result of vaccination would be the complete eradication of smallpox – the terrible scourge of the human race. The eradication of smallpox was one of the greatest successes in the history of medicine. The success of vaccination, despite the great resistance of a large part of the population, inspired many scientists to research the spread of other diseases. Among Polish scientists, the most famous was Professor Hilary Koprowski, who, while working in the USA, invented a vaccine against polio in 1950 and contributed to the rapid eradication of the disease in Poland, leading to 9 million doses of the new vaccine being sent to Polish doctors – just one year after it was introduced on the market. By now, polio has been almost completely eradicated in all corners of the globe.

When the world was optimistically entering the decade of the 1960s, which was to bring further great successes in the fight against infectious diseases, in one of the countries of Central Europe – Poland, smallpox, almost defeated, reminded of itself. The last major outbreak of smallpox in Europe was in Yugoslavia in 1972. The focus of infection turned out to be a pilgrim who had returned from the Middle East. It affected 175 people, 35 of whom died.

There is relatively little knowledge about the earliest epidemics of infectious diseases in the lands covered in this text. It seems that the plague which raged through Western Europe in the 14th century treated Central Europe, and especially the Polish lands, more gently. In older historiography there is even a claim that the first wave of the Black Death bypassed the Kingdom of Poland and Bohemia. However, this view was rejected by more recent research (Chilińska et al., 2008). It seems that the reason why this belief persisted for so long was probably the very small number of written sources on the epidemic in Poland and Bohemia (Benedictow, 2004; Mengel, 2011). As already said, the plague was mentioned in the chronicle of Jan Długosz, but his account is considered secondary and unreliable (Chilińska et al., 2008). In the second half of the century in Poland, forest cover increased, wages for workers in Krakow rose (Benedictow, 2004), and grain prices fell. The same phenomena occurred in Western European countries and were clearly linked to the epidemic and the sharp decline in population, which led to a surplus of food and therefore a fall in prices and a shortage of skilled labour and consequently an increase in wages. When the mechanism of the spread of the disease is analysed, it also seems improbable that the plague could have spared Poland, a country devoid of important natural barriers to the east and west and, moreover, surrounded on all sides by land affected by the epidemic (Benedictow, 2004). The sources also note symptoms of a social crisis related to the epidemic in Poland, i.e. flagellant processions and increased anti-Semitic sentiment (Chilińska et al., 2008). The flagellant movement was one type of reaction to the plague (Naphy & Spicer, 2004). It spread westwards from Austria and Hungary in 1348 and, after sweeping through Bohemia, central and southern Germany and Strasbourg, ended in the late summer and early autumn of 1349 in Flanders (Aberth, 2005).

In 1962, the journal *Annales* published an extensive article by the French historian Elisabeth Carpentier on research into the Black Death (Carpentier, 1962). It was illustrated with a map on which Poland and Bohemia form a green island – areas almost free of the pestilence. Despite the author's reservation about its provisional character, the map was reprinted numerous times and inspired subsequent researchers, who were probably not entirely interested in checking its credibility. Over the following decades, it found its way into multilingual studies, including those very influential and respected among historians, such as *The Black Death* by Philip Ziegler.

In 1963, Czech researcher František Graus presented evidence to support the fact that the plague struck Bohemia in 1350. The plague (or Black Death) returned repeatedly and claimed the lives of thousands of Czechs. There is therefore no question of their homeland being bypassed (Graus, 1963). In 2017 in the central Czech Republic archaeologists discovered 30 mass graves with more than 1,500 skeletons dating back to the 14th and 15th centuries. According to archaeologists, these are the graves of people who fell victim to the famine in 1318, and also the plague epidemic of 1348–1350.

The Norwegian historian Ole Benedictow, who is considered an expert on the Middle Ages and the Black Death, did not believe in the Polish miracle. His famous book – *The Black Death 1346–1353. The Complete History* – was widely commented upon by historians all over the world. It has also provoked new research on various aspects raised in his work.

If there was indeed a Polish miracle, it concerned the epidemic of 1346–1353. Meanwhile, the plague returned many times in the 14th century and beyond. And there is already rather irrefutable evidence that it did not turn out to be mild. During the reign of Casimir the Great, in 1360, the plague probably killed more than half of the Polish population, and in 1371 the Kingdom of Poland was attacked by the worst of all epidemics, *pestis puerorum* – a children's plague, characteristic of recurrences hitting the generation which had not managed to acquire short-term immunity in the previous attack. Realistically, it ceased to pose a serious threat in the 18th century. As historian Łukasz Kowalczyk argues (2019), the thesis of a green island in Central Europe is relatively new and is not based on serious historical sources but rather on a historical myth.

More importantly, the plague kept coming back over the next three centuries. At the end of the 15th century, epidemics of this disease occurred in Krakow every two or three years, or even year by year. In 1500–1750, 92 epidemics were recorded in Krakow – the largest number of any Polish city. In 1601–1650, there were 19 in Krakow and 33 in Warsaw. Later, the incidence in both cities remained at a similar level. We know about the 16th-century plagues in the lands of the Crown and Lithuania, among others, thanks to the chronicles that described trips of the rulers in search of places free from "pestilential air". Of the dozen or so infectious diseases that hit the society of the Commonwealth from the end of the Middle Ages to the 18th century, the most dangerous was the plague (Kuchowicz, 1971).

It is worth noting that in modern times epidemics went hand in hand with wars. Both of these "horsemen of the apocalypse" were favoured by chaos and the mass displacement of people. Since antiquity, epidemic diseases have had a very significant impact on the course of warfare among countries. This was due to the fact that malnourished and unwashed soldiers died of them in large numbers, and losses caused by diseases often made it impossible to conduct or complete planned campaigns. During many modern wars, the number of those killed in the battles was incomparably lower than those who died as a result of epidemics such as dysentery and typhoid fever (Zwoliński, 2020). It is not known whether part of Hungary in the mid-16th century would have fallen under Turkish rule for over 100 years if the Habsburg armies had not been attacked by typhoid fever in 1542 and 1566. The fate of the Thirty Years' War would probably have been different, too, if the fighting armies had not been decimated by infectious diseases (Karpiński, 2000). The plague, which was ravaging the armies of Sweden and the Polish Republic, was one of the main reasons for the armistice in 1629. Epidemics took a terrible toll during the wars of the mid-17th century. During the so-called Zhvania campaign during the Chmielnicki Uprising in 1653, the Crown army, which consisted of 30,000 soldiers, lost about 20,000 of them. Epidemics might also have paralysed the Battle of Vienna. "Połowa nam prawie wojska choruje na taką chorobę, która jest zarazą podobną powietrzu" ("Almost half of our army is sick with a disease which is a plague similar to the air") (Wrzesiński, 2011) – wrote Polish King Jan III Sobieski in a letter to his wife, Queen Marysieńka. Plagues also struck the devastated Polish Republic in the 18th century. In the late 1760s, the plague provided a pretext for Austria and Prussia to establish a sanitary cordon on the border with the Polish Republic. The annexations of the borderland made at that time became a prelude to the first partition of the Polish Republic in 1772.

## 1.2  Facts and myths about epidemics of infectious diseases and response to the pestilence

Infectious diseases have accompanied mankind for millennia. In every society and in every time the arrival of an epidemic was interpreted as God's punishment for people's sins (Karpiński, 2012; Kracik, 1991), also in Central Europe. The religious imagination metaphorised the plague as a hail of arrows unleashed by God (Wójcik, 2006). "The secret sins of each of us – a great misfortune, even greater – public sins, sins of the crown, nobility, the city"; it is these that cause "so many to be taken from the world" – thundered a Krakow preacher in 1723 (Dziewulski, 1723). Some tried to find other explanations for the misfortune haunting them. The Slavs, for example, believed in the god Trzybek, who spread plague air throughout the world. In the 17th century, when numerous wars ravaged the lands of the Polish Republic, the inhabitants of these lands saw the source of the plague in the huge number of unburied, decomposing corpses of people and horses left on battlefields. However, with time, especially during modern epidemics, people increasingly came to the conclusion that the infection occurred through contact with other members of the community.

Large-scale epidemics were usually preceded by various disasters and unusual weather anomalies such as warm winters, droughts and excessive rainfall. There were also strange natural phenomena, for example, large numbers of field mice, extinction of frogs and locust passages that destroyed crops. The most common symptom preceding an epidemic was usually famine as a result of the previously mentioned phenomena. Warfare also contributed to the poor physical condition of the population and the destruction of crops. It was also believed that air poisoning, which resulted in plague, was a consequence of various astronomical phenomena such as conjunction of planets,[10] meteor showers, eclipses of the Moon or the Sun and appearance of a comet (Pękacka-Falkowska, 2009).[11] Mists and winds carried away the so-called miasmas, i.e. poisonous fumes rising from the ground as a result of the phenomena, which were inhaled by people who came into contact with them. Frequent miscarriages among women and more numerous than usual births of twins were also supposed to herald the arrival of the plague. Dead fish found in the water and birds escaping from certain places also bode ill. These were widely held beliefs. These signs were treated more carefully when several of them occurred (Umiastowski, 1591).

In the Middle Ages, and this is very symptomatic, beggars, strangers, outsiders, others, vagrants, witches, Jews, people of a different race, religion or profession, or members of ethnic minorities, such as Gypsies or Tartars, were usually blamed for spreading the plague. Jews were a group that always faced accusations, which threatened harsh repression and persecution. The myth of Christians being poisoned was common. Various absurd theories arose, for example, that Jews would pour the milk of Christian women into the ears of hanged men, and it would rot there and cause epidemics (Charewiczowa, 1930). When one added to this the fact that the plague seemed to have less of an effect on Jews – most likely as a result of their somewhat more hygienic lifestyle dictated by religious precepts – the enraged mob gained an ideal enemy, which was also largely due to the desire to discredit or destroy economic competition.

During an epidemic, gravediggers were often blamed for spreading the disease on purpose so that they could have more work and earn more money. They were commonly regarded as greedy, depraved people, who killed the sick in order to seize their goods, robbed their victims and traded infected objects. For example, in some cities (e.g. Ząbkowice Śląskie in 1606, Prague in 1682, Lublin in 1711 (Klukowski, 1927)) there were trials of the so-called "smearers", i.e. gravediggers who deliberately smeared doors and doorknobs with the brains and secretions of those who died of the plague in order to spread the disease. The gang of gravediggers from Ząbkowice Śląskie was active during the plague which claimed over 2,000 inhabitants of the town, a quarter of whom were children. Marcin Koblitz, the town's chronicler and mayor, recorded that on 10 September two gravediggers were arrested for mixing and preparing poisons. During the next few days, three more suspects and three women associated with them were taken into custody (Wrzesiński, 2011). From today's point of view, the 16th–18th century smearers should be regarded as victims of epidemic fears and gloomy superstitions.

Dramatic epidemics in the 17th and 18th centuries caused increased social unrest. Accusations of deliberately causing disease became more frequent. Their victims were, among others, gravediggers, barber surgeons and witch doctors, who were suspected of wanting to make money on fake medicines or funeral arrangements. On 7 March 1711, three gravediggers were executed in Lublin, having been accused of spreading the plague. Under torture, they pleaded guilty out of a desire to make a profit. As already mentioned, the Jewish community was also accused, whose representatives were supposedly less prone to epidemic diseases. The epidemics of the 17th century also influenced the Baroque fascination with death and transience.

Not understanding the mechanisms of transmission of the plague, people tried to predict its arrival, and so in 1591 Piotr Umiastowski, a physician and philosopher educated in Bologna, in his work called *Nauka o morowym powietrzu na czwory księgi rozłożone* (Science of the plague air in four books) drew up a list of signs heralding an epidemic, which included the above-mentioned appearance of a comet, huge numbers of frogs and rapid changes in weather. The rapid putrefaction of meat exposed to the wind or the death of dogs that drank morning dew were also supposed to be signs (Wrzesiński, 2011). These were rather logical conclusions based on the belief that epidemics were caused by the "plague air".

Regardless of the country, throughout Central Europe the news of the approaching epidemic caused widespread panic. The royal court (Bończak, 1968; Lernet, 1817; Ptaśnik, 1903) and representatives of the secular and clerical elites (Lileyko, 1984; Vorbeck-Lettow, 1968; Walawender, 1932) fled from the threatened areas. In Poland, for example, royal exodus, or rather royal flight, was once very frequent, especially during the long reign of Sigismund I the Old of the Jagiellonian dynasty. Władysław Jagiełło, Kazimierz Jagiellończyk, Zygmunt August and Zygmunt III Waza fled. One of the most visible effects of the approaching plague was therefore the migration of people from the threatened city or area. Panic also gripped the representatives of urban commoners. The approaching plague also caused doctors and many lower-ranking officials, including executioners, to flee (Karpiński, 2000). The recognition of flight as the most effective form of protection against the plague was, of course, very old. It was already recommended by the famous Greek physician Hippocrates and another father of medicine, Galen (Kracik, 2012). Thus, the first and common way to avoid infection during an epidemic was to flee the area affected by the plague. Everyone who could afford it fled, often contributing to the spread of the epidemic. In some cases, all the town officials with the mayor at the head fled. The first to flee to the countryside were, of course, the wealthy, who had the means and opportunities to survive a long time away from home. The poor, who lived from day to day, remained in the city. Not infrequently, in desperation, people took refuge in the forests, but the living conditions there were very difficult. The sought-after oases were not invariably good for health. For example, in 1451 Cardinal Zbigniew Oleśnicki fled from an epidemic through forests and swamps (Kracik, 1991). Many of those fleeing became infected or died on the way. Many carried the plague into the countryside.

When the Black Death was coming back to Wawel, the town hall was wondering what to do so that the depopulated city would not be given away to the villains because of the mass exodus. After all, in the autumn of 1622 night-time plundering of dwellings began. During the epidemics, there was the strengthening of guards, who were supposed not only to see to the segregation of the healthy and the sick but also to guard the houses against robbery, as it was explicitly stated in the publications of 1543, 1691 or 1707 (Kracik, 1991).

Two types of isolation can be distinguished during an epidemic: voluntary and forced. Voluntary isolation was chosen by wealthy people, who having heard of the approaching plague made large stocks and locked themselves and their families up in their properties, leaving them only after the plague had stopped. They baked their own bread, brewed their own beer and used the resources they had accumulated before the epidemic. Forced isolation of the sick has accompanied epidemics since time immemorial. People quickly realised that the disease was spreading from person to person and tried to avoid direct contact. In the 14th century, quarantine became widespread – Italian: *quaranta giorni* = forty days, i.e. a 40-day isolation of healthy people newly arrived in a given place in order to observe whether they had any symptoms of the disease.[12] During the plague epidemic, many European sources mention the forced isolation of the infected and their fellow inhabitants confined to their own homes. Where at least one case of the disease was found, the authorities ordered a quarantine. Doors were boarded up from the outside and marked with a white cross. Municipal guards were placed in front of the door (Drążkowska, 2008). Whoever left such a household or concealed the illness or death of a family member ended up in the gallows.

Undoubtedly, both great and local pestilences paralysed the already weak institutions of the Polish state. Sources often mention the suspension of the work of courts and tribunals. A completely exceptional measure was the delay of key state events, including funerals. The plague in Krakow in 1599 delayed the funeral of Queen Anna Habsburg by a year.

In the large cities of the Polish Republic, after city officials fled from the plague, a "plague mayor" was elected to lead the city. His first move was usually to issue the "plague regulations", as well as to significantly increase the salaries of those who worked with the infected, i.e. the so-called "air service", for example, barber surgeons, stewards, nurses, hospital and municipal kitchen workers, gravediggers, watchmen and city guards, alms collectors, dogcatchers and cleaners of infected houses. A famous plague ("air") mayor was a Varsovian – pharmacist, Łukasz Drewno. He distinguished himself by being the first to introduce isolation rooms for the sick. His description of the plague epidemic in Warsaw in 1624–1625, which has survived to the present day, is an excellent example of order regulations at the time of the epidemic and the resulting developments. He established a sanitary police in order to maintain order in the city. The burial of the dead was carried out by porters-diggers dressed in red gowns with a black cross on their chests. A similar outfit was worn by expellers, who removed potential pestilence spreaders from the city. The sick were transported to a field hospital (lazaret) on an island in the Vistula, near today's Citadel. Food and medicine were given to them by the diggers, who also took the bodies of the dead. Windows and doors in the infected houses were boarded up. Parts of the city where the plague was found were cordoned off with palisades.

A black cross was placed there as a warning sign. Prisoners were forced to clean the streets, which were drowning in mud and waste. The bodies of the victims were covered with lye and buried outside the town. Guards were placed at the graves to prevent thieves from digging them up and relatives from taking the bodies to church cemeteries. There were threats of flogging and even the gallows for looting the clothes of the dead.

As in Warsaw, other cities in Central Europe, such as Krakow and Lviv, had special rules and regulations during the plague. Particular emphasis was placed on those who buried epidemic victims. Gravediggers were always obliged to wear distinctive clothing, most often, unlike in Warsaw, these were black coats marked with white crosses. As in the rest of Europe, gravediggers had to signal their presence with a bell attached to corpse-carrying carts (Wrzesiński, 2008). They were paid a solid wage. Prisoners and convicts were forced to do the work if there were not enough people willing to do it. However, due to the loss of many jobs, there were usually enough people willing to take care of the work. During the plague, various occupational specialisations arose that had never been seen before: corpse seekers, plague mothers feeding the infants of the dead, cleaners of infected houses and poverty expellers. The plague disturbed the previously existing social hierarchy and opened up unprecedented opportunities for socio-economic advancement for people from the poor and marginalised groups.

And if someone wanted to feel truly safe, they reached for the fire. Items that were commonly believed to provide a favourable environment for the plague – above all wood and fur – were burnt. Clothing had to be aired out in the cold and anything of lesser value had to be burnt (Kracik, 1991).

Łukasz Drewno survived the epidemic, but his daughter, son-in-law and three grandchildren died during the plague (Baranowski, 1915). The plague killed 15–20% of Warsaw inhabitants. After these events, in the 17th century, the plague returned to Warsaw eight more times. A memento of the epidemic of 1708 is the Warsaw walking pilgrimage to Jasna Góra. The first 200 pilgrims set out in July 1711 to ask the Mother of God to save the city.

A very important role was played by gravediggers (Polish: kopacze), who, in addition to a salary supplement, were entitled to accommodation outside the city walls, food and booze. The already mentioned "poverty expellers" were also appointed – as a new function of city officials – whose task was to drive out potential plague spreaders from the city, i.e. beggars, prostitutes, homeless people and "loose people". For example, in July 1543, beggars and scoundrels were to leave the city immediately (Walawender, 1957). Antisocial, dirty and giving off a bad odour, they were considered potential pestilence sowers, and on top of that they would have to be fed in the closed city. One of the duties of the guards was to watch over quarantined houses and supply food to inhabitants. Those who wanted to enter the city, , merchants, had to present a so-called health passport. This was a certificate issued by the city authorities or parishes from the mid-17th century onwards, stating that the persons concerned were coming from a plague-free area. A sick person caught trying to enter a city was liable to a death penalty.

It was forbidden to spill waste in the streets or to keep cattle or poultry in farmyards. Rubbish and manure were to be urgently cleaned up from the streets, and pigs and other animals were not to be allowed to run free. Pets were ordered to be disposed of. Anti-plague manuals recommended banishing dogs and cats or killing them, as their fur was a breeding ground for plague. Butchers were also obliged to slaughter animals outside the city. When further epidemics broke out, these and similar ordinances were repeated, with reminders to remove mud and waste [*Prawa, przywileje i statuta...* 1890–1910]. The regularity of these reminders makes one doubt that good habits were acquired. In Krakow in 1712, following foreign models, it was decided to establish a tax on cleaning and to set up an equivalent of today's municipal cleaning company. However, two years later a reminder of the obligation to keep order in front of one's own tenement house makes one doubt whether the equivalent of the municipal cleaning company was adopted in the early 18th century (Kracik, 2012).

Lavish family celebrations and feasts with music and dance were forbidden. Staging of plays was forbidden. In order to restrict public gatherings, schools, courts and offices were closed. For example, in July 1543, the magistrate of Krakow ordered the closure of inns and public baths and banned free sale of fruit and vegetables, as well as trade in old goods (Kracik, 1991). Only churches usually remained open and full of worshippers during epidemics. However, special regulations were also issued for the clergy during the plague. The burial of the sick was forbidden in churches and church cemeteries. Plague cemeteries were set up outside the town and mass graves were dug during large waves of deaths. The family of the deceased was not allowed to take part in the burial, only the town gravediggers, who brought the corpses in carts, usually at night. Bodies were also buried in the fields and forests or drowned in rivers and lakes. Many were afraid to report the death of a household member, knowing that the living would be quarantined or taken to a field hospital. In order to raise funds for the fight against the plague and to maintain the field hospitals, the authorities organised various fund-raisers and collections; they passed extraordinary taxes on the infected areas, the so-called airways, and took out loans from foundations and private individuals. The city budget during the epidemics was also supported by the proceeds from city fines, imposed on people who did not observe the epidemic regulations, and legacies of the dead, although those usually went to the church budget, as well as the so-called "ransom payments" paid by the family in exchange for placing their relative in the field hospital for the plagued. Special plague isolation buildings were built outside city walls. For example, in Krakow, during the plague of 1652, there were three types of them: for patients infected with the plague, for people in contact with the sick, and for high-risk groups: paupers, beggars, etc.

The sick were cared for in municipal hospitals, but when there was a lack of space, buildings far outside the city walls were usually set aside for the sick. These were not places of treatment but rather "places of isolation, preparation for death, dying and burial" (Kracik, 1991).

The 16th-, 17th- and 18th-century epidemics also left lasting traces in architecture, urban planning and sculpture. In the countries of the former Habsburg Monarchy, including Bohemia, Austria and Hungary, the erection of the so-called "plague columns" was popular for centuries. They were erected in representative parts of the city as a thanksgiving votive offering from the religious people for the salvation of the community from the plague or another aggressive infectious disease. They can still be seen today, for example, in Budapest or Olomouc (see Prucek, 1991).[13] In the Hungarian capital, the experience of the plague is recalled, for example, by the Baroque Holy Trinity Column located on Trinity Square, opposite the famous Matthias Church. The column commemorates the victims of the two Black Death epidemics that swept through Europe in 1691 and 1709. Only five years after the recapture of Buda from the Turks by united Christian armies in 1686, in addition to rebuilding the destroyed and depopulated city, the new inhabitants had to face another major challenge: the plague. The inhabitants took a solemn oath to erect a column as an act of gratitude if they survived the epidemic.[14]

Individual anti-plague practices included: living in stables with horses, as the protective effect of horse manure and breath was believed to be present; incensing dwellings with herbs, juniper, amber, sulphur, resin and tobacco; limiting sexual contact; lubricating oneself with vinegar and camphor or rose vodka; avoiding overeating and sweets; carrying protective amulets; drinking a spoonful of one's own urine every morning (Pękacka-Falkowska, 2009); keeping a stinking goat in the house; bloodletting and enemas; having a cheerful disposition, remaining optimistic and avoiding strong emotions (Karpiński, 2000); chewing angelica and orange peel; eating large amounts of garlic and onions, nuts and radishes; avoiding fogs and warm south-west winds, which spread the plague air; washing the inside walls with vinegar-dampened sheets, sprinkling the floors with fragrances and sprinkling the beds with vinegar; singing aloud, shouting, reading aloud, driving away roaring cattle to ward off the plague; carrying a sponge soaked in vinegar or spices, chewing herbs, rubbing them on the nostrils and the area around the heart; firing cannons (Podgórscy, 2005) and rifles to dry the air and rid it of pathogenic miasmas; making the sign of the cross on the lips while yawning; burning horse manure, bones and animal horns to incense the house and prevent the entry of deadly miasmas; eating easily digestible food, well-baked bread, flying fowl, fish from rivers, dried fruit and curdled milk; wearing precious stones on the naked body (topaz, emerald, sapphire, jasper), as well as wearing pearls, amber, ivory, mercury in hazelnut shell, powdered frog, a bottle with a mixture of arsenic and camphor, goat liver, unicorn horn, etc. (Rożek, 2016; Wrzesiński, 2011); avoiding baths and the use of soap, as the enlarged pores of the skin make it easier for the germs to penetrate the body; the use of various paramedical products: scabious (powdered herbs with wine, honey and opium) (Kracik, 2012), vinegar of the four thieves (wine vinegar in which basil, wormwood, rue, sage were soaked for 12 days), Ruff's pills (myrrh, saffron and aloe) (Brodzicki, 2000), St. Roch's pills made of clay, tar root, scorpion oil, tobacco, and many other ingredients; wearing of masks with a beak on the face, which contained herbs and oils to prevent contagion; and prayer and the direct touch of relics of patron saints against the plague air. Many extraordinary anti-plague properties were attributed to pebbles found in the bladder, kidneys or stomach of various animals, which were called bezoars (Jarczykowa, 2015; Umiastowski, 1591).

## 1.3 The state and epidemics of infectious diseases from a historical perspective

Attempts to stop the plague or to reduce its effects caused both monarchs, as well as ecclesiastical institutions and municipal governments to become active. It was up to the latter to fight the plague properly, and this was led in towns either by officials of special Health Offices or by so-called "air mayors". In both cases, direct care of the infected was provided by doctors and barber surgeons, as well as "air guards", nurses and diggers recruited from the urban poor. Another important task was to provide material and medical aid to as many people in need as possible. This included the plagued as well as the impoverished and starving representatives of the folk and the poor. Some elements of interpersonal solidarity can be observed in actions of this kind, which manifested itself in the contribution of private donations to the so-called "plague funds" (Karpiński, 2000).

The first interventions of the state in general in the area of health took place precisely in connection with infectious diseases, and this intervention was to increase with time. It was up to the municipal authorities to deal with sewage and latrines, to drain the used water, to supervise establishments harmful to health, to control the sanitation of foodstuffs and so on. In the 17th century, in order to realise the extent of the epidemic, the English administration introduced a compulsory register of deaths and births in parishes – thus initiating sanitary statistics and demographic studies. In the 18th century, the king's administrators in the French provinces were obliged to inform the metropolitan authorities of cases of rash fevers, the plague, cattle diseases and famines (Ruffié & Sournia, 1996).

From the end of the 17th century in Western Europe increasing interference of the central authorities in health and hygiene issues of the population of the subordinated territory could be observed, which eventually led in the 18th century to the total control of this sector of social life by the state. If one takes a closer look at Central Europe, for example, at the Polish Republic, analogous processes were much slower and clearly lagged behind the West (Pękacka-Falkowska, 2009). As far as anti-plague activity is concerned, on the territory of the Polish Republic, regular air services were developed only in the large cities of Royal Prussia, which already in the 17th century adopted German solutions in this matter (Karpiński, 2000). On the remaining territory of the state there were only ad hoc institutions, the management of which was entrusted to ad hoc elected air stewards (Charewiczowa, 1930).

On the territory of the Polish Republic, the interference of the central authorities in the issues of health and hygiene of the population, including the assumption of control over anti-plague actions, i.e. the creation of the first central institutions established to fight the plague, did not take place until the 1770s (Wrzesiński, 2008). The breakthrough was connected with nationwide actions undertaken by the cabinet of King Stanisław August Poniatowski to quell the spreading plague, and with the establishment of a central decision-making centre – the Permanent Council (see Srogosz, 1997). The end of the plague in Europe coincided with global actions taken by various states. In the Polish Republic, the reign of the last King was characterised by the efforts of the enlightened elites to modernise the state, create a modern administration and a strong and modern army, and develop the economy, education and culture. Publicists and doctors of the time recognised the danger of depopulation, as well as poor sanitary and health conditions. The structures of the state directed all possible forces and resources to suppress the plague: the army, treasury administration, diplomatic service, doctors, feldshers, as well as funds commensurate with the budget. In the conditions of lagging behind in terms of civilisation development of the Polish Republic, it was quite a feat, and in some respects, according to Tadeusz Srogosz, Polish anti-epidemic solutions could have become an example for other countries, perhaps due to the scale of the threat.

Until then, the protection of the population against epidemics rested solely on the shoulders of the local municipal government. The approaching danger to the town was announced by notices from the town councils and by the clergy at mass (Charytoniuk, 1985; Salmonowicz, 1983). In people's minds, even in Saxon times, it was mainly the city and the urban space around it that was perceived as a dangerous area, a kind of "cesspit of humanity" (Popiołek, 2016).

It is worth mentioning that, when talking about contemporary Central Europe from a historical perspective and state action in response to epidemics, it was in the Austrian Empire, for example, that an effective sanitary cordon was established in 1739. More than 4,000 army troops were henceforth permanently stationed on the borders of Slavonia, Croatia and Transylvania and along the Danube. They consisted of flying brigades to ensure the tightness of the borders. Anyone who tried to slip through them was shot at without mercy (Naphy & Spicer, 2004).

It should not be forgotten that, as in modern times, charitable initiatives in the past by the nation's elite were also of great importance in the fight against epidemics. For example, at the beginning of the Great War, Prince Adam Sapieha, Bishop of Krakow, created a sanitary section that was composed mainly of medical students (Urban, 2016). They were given the task of reaching the smallest villages in Galicia in order to inoculate the local peasants. These measures might have saved up to 3 million inhabitants of the region. In turn, vaccination against typhus reduced the risk of a typhus epidemic during the Second World War. The vaccines produced in Rudolf

Weigl's famous laboratory in Lviv (Złotorzycka, 1998) were smuggled into the ghettos where typhus took the heaviest toll. It should be noted that in Poland, regular vaccinations with Weigl's vaccine began as early as 1934, inoculating 8,000 people, mainly among the sanitary staff and those most exposed to infection (Ciesielska, 2015).

Analysing the initiatives of Central European countries towards the epidemic, it is worth recalling the following example: on 1 August 1919, in view of the huge number of typhus cases, the Central Anti-Typhus Committee was established in Poland. It consisted of the Minister of Public Health – Witold Chodźko as Chairman, his deputy, the head of the American Sanitary Mission, the head of the English Mission of the British Society of Friends, as well as ministry officials and appointed delegates. The battle plan was given the name "The Great National Cleansing Action". It provided for sanitation, i.e. the careful cleansing of towns where typhoid fever had been reported by cleaning houses, streets, cleansing sewers and toilets, including their dumping with slaked lime, and disposing of rubbish and waste. The population was to be bathed and their hair was to be cut, and clothing was to be deloused. All the Committee's actions were to be consulted on an ongoing basis with the sanitary chiefs of the relevant sections, as warfare was still ongoing in eastern Poland. However, the effects of the Committee's actions were not satisfactory, so in March 1920, on the motion of the Minister of Public Health, the Commander-in-Chief appointed a professor from the Jagiellonian University's Faculty of Medicine as the Chief Extraordinary Commissioner for Combating Epidemics and assigned three extraordinary commissioners to assist him. The Committee was replaced by the Supreme Sanitary Council, which was to play a coordinating role in the field of social hygiene. The coordinated actions of the Chief Commissioner and the Sanitary Council contributed to the reduction of disease outbreaks in the eastern territories. Parallel to his internal activities, Minister Chodźko sought help in London. In the summer of 1919, the British Society of Friends sent to Poland a small group of people prepared to fight the disease (Ciesielska, 2015). The American Red Cross also came to Poland's aid in the spring of 1919, sending a 50-strong delegation of workers (Strong, 1920 and 378 wagons of donations (clothing, food, medicines, medical equipment and equipment for pest control). In addition, the mission financially supported the activities of the League of Red Cross Societies, which was established by the League of Nations in May, by donating USD 400,000 for a planned expedition to Poland. President Wilson was asked to help Poland by the President of the American Relief Administration, Herbert Hoover, and as a result an American team of the APRE (The American-Polish Relief Expedition) (Trask, 1983) went to Poland. Unfortunately, American-Polish cooperation brought mutual accusations of incompetence and unwillingness. In reality, the APRE mission brought measurable benefits. It was one of many actions limiting the epidemic in Poland. The action covered a total of 311,374 people (72,731 homes). Four mobile American columns disinfected 19,400 people, while the British Society cleansed 2,800 houses and

15,860 people (Strong, 1920). In order to prevent infected lice from penetrating further into the country, a sanitary cordon was established along Poland's eastern border. Anyone crossing the border posts had to undergo compulsory delousing.

It should be noted that one of the first pieces of legislation that came into being after Poland regained independence was the Sanitary Act of 1919, which required the authorities to contain epidemics of infectious diseases, to supervise safe water and food, but also hospitals. It was also then that recommendations were made on vaccination and sanitisation of water. In the 20th century, it was, of course, mainly doctors who fought epidemics, but the role of law enforcement, for example, was also important. And so, it is worth noting the role the Polish police played in fighting the Spanish flu. At that time, police officers were used by the state administration for various activities outside their primary tasks. A document preserved in the Archives of New Records in Warsaw features the tasks of the police in the city of Lviv. Section 8 reads that the tasks of the police include intervening in public disasters, fires, floods, epidemics, sudden collapses and suicide attempts.

Analysing the state's behaviour in the face of an epidemic from a historical perspective, it is worth looking through the lens of the last time smallpox appeared in Central Europe – in Poland, in Wrocław, in 1963. The disease was brought in May by Bonifacy Jedynak, an officer of the Security Service, who came back from Asia. Ninety-nine people fell ill, mainly medical staff, and seven died.[15] The city was paralysed for several weeks and cut off from the rest of the country by a sanitary cordon. Ninety-eight per cent of the Wrocław population was vaccinated, as compulsory vaccination of all inhabitants was introduced. Evaders faced a fine or three months' imprisonment. Refusal of treatment and causing the risk of infecting others carried the penalty of up to 15 years in prison (Rosalak, 2020). Two thousand people who had contact with the sick were isolated. Posters were put up in the city: "Let's greet without shaking hands". Doorknobs and handrails were covered with bandages soaked in chloramine, and the sale of bread in the self-service system was abolished. Swimming pools were closed during that hot summer (Sobków, 2000). Company vehicles were requisitioned, among other things, for the sanitary transport of those who had been sent to the isolation centres. They were taken unexpectedly at night, as some had fled their homes during the day. The state of the epidemic lasted from 17 July to 19 September. Nevertheless, smallpox spread to five other provinces without causing an epidemic there. WHO predicted that the epidemic would last for two years, with 2,000 people falling ill and 200 dying. However, it died out after 25 days from its detection. It was only after the epidemic threat was cancelled that the whole of Poland was able to learn what life was really like for the citizens of Wrocław in the city affected by the infection.

When an epidemic of smallpox broke out, the city was sealed off and entry and exit were controlled by the militia. The disease wreaked havoc in

Wrocław, reaching various towns in Lower Silesia and the Opole voivodship and threatening others. The circumstances in which smallpox appeared in Wrocław, as well as the inconvenient date of its diagnosis in mid-July –22nd July was the date on which the pompous celebrations of the national holiday were planned – contributed to the fact that the city authorities concealed the enormity of the threat. This state of affairs was aggravated by the lack of trained medical staff who would know the methods of fighting this deadly disease, as well as the complete unpreparedness of the state administration in this area. There was no adequate law on combating epidemics in Poland, and the one in force from 1935 did not meet the requirements. Neither were any detailed regulations drawn up, such as orders or instructions concerning isolation rooms, organisation of epidemiological hospitals or procedures for dealing with the sick and people in contact with them. Above all, adequate stocks of smallpox vaccine, which was the main and most effective tool in the fight against the epidemic, were not secured. In this situation the effort of the front-line medical personnel was enormous. Considering also the state of the Polish economy in the 1960s, one had to take into consideration great difficulties in the organisation of transport, limited access to disinfectants and personal protection for health workers and means of telecommunications.

The results of the work of the health service were already visible in mid-August, when there was a systematic decrease in the number of sick people. Over 2.5 million people were vaccinated in Lower Silesia. In Wrocław alone about 1,400 were isolated in specially prepared buildings, and the isolation period lasted 21 days. In addition, several facilities were quarantined. In September 1963, after the epidemic had died down, the local party authorities made many proposals, which failed to be implemented on several important points, such as the construction of a modern infectious diseases hospital in the city.

## 1.4 Conclusions

Pestilences – epidemics and pandemics – have always accompanied humanity. Some of them contributed to a deep crisis of empires; others provided an opportunity to catch up with the civilisational gap between less and more developed societies.

According to Wolfgang Reinhard, the four main plagues haunting European society were: wars of aggression, civil wars, famine and epidemics (Reinhardt, 2006). The same happened in the territories of the countries that make up contemporary Central Europe. These major epidemics not only wipe out populations but also bring about economic,[16] political, social, psychological, cultural and religious changes. Epidemics of infectious diseases were one of the main factors behind the economic collapse and crisis of the Polish–Lithuanian Commonwealth, which had a significant impact on the weakening of the Polish state in the second half of the 17th century and its collapse in the following century (Karpiński, 2000). Epidemics undoubtedly hampered the functioning of state institutions (see Bończak, 1968; Gąsiorowski, 1839; Giedroyć, 1899; Kronika Pawła Piaseckiego, 1870), the judiciary (Namaczyńska, 1937; Walawender, 1932), and the disorganisation of church structures and offices (Wyrobisz, 1999). For example, the Black Death brought an increase in wages for craftsmen and hired workers. The decline in population meant that anyone with the strength and skills to do the job was literally worth their weight in gold. A less desirable effect of the epidemic was, for example, the closure of the city's baths. In later times, the outbreak of subsequent epidemics resulted in the acceleration of work on antidotes and the improvement of general principles of hygiene. For example, in the Polish lands, on the one hand, epidemics of infectious diseases had a negative impact on the functioning of Polish education, but on the other hand, they became a stimulus for the development of 16th/18th century medicine, especially epidemiology. In this respect, eminent Polish physicians, especially lecturers and professors of the Academy of Krakow, easily kept pace with the then European authorities from Western Europe (Piotrowski, 1996). Of course, not all the changes were positive. Many epidemics affected Jews, who were accused of infecting wells or performing witchcraft against Christians, and pogroms were organised. It is true though that in the 16th–18th centuries pogroms on the scale as in the mid-14th century were not repeated in the Polish lands (Jankowski, 1990). However, Jews were always the main scapegoat, especially in the 17th and 18th centuries. Certainly the fear of Black Death influenced the growth of xenophobia and superstitiousness.

One way or another, however, epidemics have pushed humanity forward, changed the way we look at reality. They have also been a catalyst for economic change. After all, the "plagues make history",[17] since they are the event-matrices: their occurrence becomes as much a teratologic obstacle in the process of the structural development of a society or a state as it is a catalyst for that development (Pękacka-Falkowska, 2009). It is hard not to agree with Michel Foucault's view that it was the defence against the plague that was at the genesis of the emergence of 19th-century disciplinary devices and practices that continue to this day. He wrote: "The plague-stricken town, traversed throughout with hierarchy, surveillance, observation, writing; the town immobilised by the functioning of an extensive power that bears in a distinct way over all individual bodies – this is the utopia of the perfectly governed city" (Foucault, 1998).

In this chapter, it can be clearly seen that the experience of epidemics in Central European states in the past proves that, as today, the inhabitants of the states needed elites, both secular and clerical, while these were absent, fled, were preoccupied with themselves or did not know how to respond or showed no interest whatsoever. In the past and at present alike, states and their inhabitants have needed authorities, and yet, because of their scarcity, home-grown and self-proclaimed shamans, witches, preachers, pseudo-scientists or feldschers were believed and real scholars or experts were difficult to believe and their voices could not break through the information noise.

Witchcraft and belief in various miracle workers were widespread. Many tried to make a business out of the plague and found a lucrative way of life. Out of fear, people believed in superstitions and looked for scapegoats, the so-called "plague sowers", because it was easier that way, and unfortunately this has not changed. Outbreaks of infectious diseases have always resulted in stigmatisation and a search for those to blame. This is due to a sense of threat, disinformation, and panicky social reactions. Without access to science and reliable knowledge, people believed only in God's help. The fight against the epidemic was believed to be a prayer, a promised pilgrimage, a funded plague column. One can also see how, from a historical perspective, epidemics and pandemics were part of the political game, both within and among countries, or that despite centuries of experience, the fight against the disease is still based on isolation, often forced, quarantine, closure of specific sectors of the economy, banning gatherings, etc., sanitary cordons of the army and police, and, later, compulsory vaccinations. The management of restrictions in Central Europe was, as it is today, chaotic. This is due, among other things, to the fact that those in power do not make much use of expert knowledge, are attached to an excessive belief in their own infallibility and their actions are of an ad hoc nature.

The final conclusion is that, historically, the state, particularly at the central level, was too late in taking up the fight against infectious disease epidemics. Perhaps, then, historical experience teaches us that the centre of gravity needs to be shifted – let local authorities fight infectious diseases as they did centuries ago, with the support of central government and international cooperation. Perhaps history speaks in favour of a decentralised response.

## Notes

1 An entry for 1348 reads: "The great plague, which spread death throughout the Kingdom of Poland, ravaged not only Poland, but also Hungary, Bohemia, Denmark, France, Germany and almost all Christian and barbarian countries".
2 In Old Poland, the colloquial language of our ancestors abounded in many interchangeable names for the disease referred to as the plague today: *mór, przymorek, czarna śmierć* (Black Death), *złe powietrze* (bad air), *morowe powietrze* (plague air), *zaraza morowa, aura pestifera, pestilencia.*
3 The major European epidemics occurred in: 1449, 1460, 1473, 1482–1483, 1521–1527, 1545–1547, 1562–1566, 1575–1582, 1602, 1622, 1625, 1652–1653, 1668–1670 (cf.: Rosalak, 2020).
4 A reasonably reliable estimate of the number of dead in Prussia is 300,000 victims between 1709 and 1713.
5 Or the starving fever (Ciesielska, 2015).
6 In Russia, after the outbreak of the 1917 revolution, 25 million citizens fell ill with typhus.
7 (Against the "Spanish" of the prophylactic company [in] Illustrated Daily Courier 1918, 201, 4). Przeciw „hiszpance" znakomity środek profilaktyczny [w:] Ilustrowany Kurier Codzienny 1918, 201, 4.
8 Z.T., Hiszpanka [w:] Kurier Poznański 1918, 259, 3.
9 Among American Indians it could have reached 90% (see Aberth, 2012).

10  A conjunction of two planets under the sign of a third, e.g. Jupiter, Saturn, Mars was considered particularly fatal for humans (Rutkowska-Płachcińska, 1978).

11  Comets were also blamed for poisoning the air with deadly venoms (see Sokół, 1960).

12  The first quarantine for arriving merchants was applied by the Republic of Venice and the Republic of Ragusa (Dubrovnik).

13  In Olomouc, the Marian Plague Column is a striking monument located in the Lower Square. It is a plague column topped with a statue of the Virgin Mary and erected in connection with the tragic Black Death epidemic that took place in the city between 1713 and 1715. The situation was so serious that the town was sealed off and surrounded by troops. The column was erected between 1716 and 1724 to express the gratitude of the townspeople for having survived or escaped this terrible disease.

14  The first pillar was erected between 1700 and 1706 in memory of the victims of the plague of 1691. In 1709 there was a second major outbreak of the plague, after which the Buda Council decided to erect a much larger and more imposing Holy Trinity Column. The sculptors were Philipp Ungleich and Anton Hörger, and the new column was completed in 1713.

15  The first victim was Ilona Kowalczyk, daughter of the maid cleaning the isolation room where the officer was staying. The next victims were the maid's son and the doctor from whom the maid sought advice (Rosalak, 2020). The ward maid herself underwent the abortive form of the disease with a mild course.

16  It is worth mentioning the collapse of urban trade and crafts caused by the plague, the impediments to foreign trade, the dying out of the rural population, the shrinking of state revenues and the rapid pauperisation of large sections of society.

17  The author of the slogan is the American historian, William McNeill (1976).

# References

Aberth, J. (2005). *The Black Death: The Great Mortality of 1348–1350. A Brief History with Documents*. Boston: Bedford/St. Martin's.

Aberth, J. (2012). *Spektakle masowej śmierci. Plagi, zarazy, epidemie*. Warszawa: Świat Książki.

Adams F. (1886). *The Genuine Works of Hippocrates*. New York: William Wood.

Allen, A. (2016). *Fantastyczne laboratorium doktora Weigla. Lwowscy uczeni, tyfus i walka z Niemcami*. Wołowiec: Wydawnictwo Czarne.

Baranowski, I. (1915). *Z dziejów rodów patrycyuszowskich miasta Starej Warszawy*. Warszawa: Towarzystwo Miłośników Historyi.

Benedictow, O.J. (2004). *The Black Death 1346–1353. The Complete History*. Woodbridge: The Boydell Press.

Berner, W. (2008). Z dziejów walki z ostrymi chorobami zakaźnymi w Polsce po I wojnie światowej – do 1920 r. (z uwzględnieniem wielkich miast). *Przegląd Epidemiologiczny*, 62.

Bończak, J. (1968). Dur brzuszny w armiach na przestrzeni wieków. *Lekarz Wojskowy RXLIV*, 12.

Brodzicki, C. (2000). Morowe powietrze w XVI wieku w Polsce i przeciwdziałanie jemu, zalecane przez Marcina Ruffusa z Wałcza, cyrulika i medyka łomżyńskiego. *Analecta R. 9(1)*.

Brown, J. (2019). *Grypa. Sto lat walki*. Kraków: Wydawnictwo Uniwersytetu Jagiellońskiego.

Brydak, L.B. (2008). *Grypa. Pandemia grypy: mit czy realne zagrożenie?* Warszawa: Oficyna Wydawnicza RYTM.

Carpentier, E. (1962). Autour de la peste noire. Famines et épidémies dans l'histoire du XIVe siècle. *Annales ESC*, 17(6).

Charewiczowa, Ł. (1930). *Klęska zaraz w dawnym Lwowie*. Wydawca: Nakł. Towarzystwa Miłośników Przeszłości Lwowa.

Charytoniuk, J. (1985). Walka z epidemią dżumy w Elblągu na początku XVIII wieku. *Rocznik Elbląski*, 10.

Chilińska, A., Zawadzka, U., & Sołtysiak, A. (2008). Pandemia dżumy w latach 1348–1379 na terenach Królestwa Polskiego. Model epidemiologiczny i źródła historyczne. In W. Dzieduszycki, & J. Wrzesiński (Eds.), *Epidemie, klęski, wojny*. Funeralia Lednickie – Spotkanie 10. Poznań: Wydawnictwo SNAP.

Ciesielska, M. (2015). *Tyfus – groźny zabójca i cichy sprzymierzeniec*. Warszawa: Stowarzyszenie EKOSAN.

Collier, R. (1974). *The Plague of the Spanish Lady*. London: Macmillan.

Colwell, R.R. (1996). Global Climate and Infectious Disease: The Cholera Paradigm. *Science*, 274(5295).

Drążkowska, A. (2008). Kilka uwag na temat sposobów walki z dżumą w XVII i XVIII wieku. In W. Dzieduszycki, & J. Wrzesiński (Eds.), *Epidemie, klęski, wojny*. Funeralia Lednickie – Spotkanie 10. Poznań: Wydawnictwo SNAP.

Dziewulski, M. (1723). Hamulec gniewu Bożego, Beatissima V. Maria de Gratiis, to jak łask Boskich pełna Matka Łaskawa Najświętsza Marya Panna. Kraków, fol. Fv.

Faron, B. (2021). *Jak przetrwać zarazy w dawnej Polsce*. Kraków: Wydawnictwo Astra.

Foucault, M. (1998). *Nadzorować i karać. Narodziny więzienia*. Warszawa: Aletheia.

Gambal-Różańska, B. (2008). Występowanie epidemii ospy prawdziwej na świecie od czasów starożytnych po współczesne. *Medycyna Nowożytna*, 15(1–2).

Gąsiorowski, L. (1839). *Zbiór wiadomości do historii sztuki lekarskiej w Polsce od czasów najdawniejszych aż do najnowszych*. Vol. I. Poznań: drukarnia K.A. Pompejusza Gilewska – Dubis J.

Giedroyć, F. (1899). *Mór w Polsce w wiekach ubiegłych. Zarys historyczny*. Warszawa: L. Szkaradziński.

Górski, A. (2008). Wspomnienie zarazy 1709 roku w zachowanych artefaktach epigraficznych. In W. Dzieduszycki, & J. Wrzesiński (Eds.), *Epidemie, klęski, wojny*. Funeralia Lednickie – Spotkanie 10. Poznań: Wydawnictwo SNAP.

Graus, F. (1963). Autour de la peste noire au XIVe siècle en Bohême. *Annales ESC*, 18(4).

Jankowski, J. (1990). *Epidemiologia historyczna polskiego średniowiecza*. Kraków: Zarząd Główny Polskiego Towarzystwa Schweitzerowskiego.

Jarczykowa, M. (2015). "Powietrzna zaraza" w Wielkim Księstwie Litewskim w ujęciu Walentego Bartoszewskiego i Piotra Kochlewskiego. In M. Jarczykowa, B. Mazurkowa, S. Dąbrowski (Eds.), *Świat bliski i świat daleki w staropolskich przestrzeniach*. Katowice: Uniwersytet Śląski.

Jasiński K. (2019). *Śmierć przypłynęła na okrętach*, Rp.pl Historia z 23 listopada 2019 (Accessed: 16 December 2021).

Karpiński, A. (2000). *W walce z niewidzialnym wrogiem*. Warszawa: Wydawnictwo Neriton, Instytut Historii PAN.

Karpiński, A. (2012). Epidemie w Rzeczypospolitej od XVI do XVIII wieku. In E. Kizik (Ed.), *Dżuma, ospa, cholera. W trzechsetletnią rocznicę wielkiej epidemii w Gdańsku i na ziemiach Rzeczypospolitej w latach 1708–1711*. Materiały z konferencji naukowej zorganizowanej przez Muzeum Historyczne Miasta Gdańska i Instytut Historii PAN w dniach 21–22 maja 2009 roku.

Klukowski, Z. (1927). Sprawa o szerzenie dżumy w Lublinie w r. 1711. *AHFM*, 6(1).

Kowalczyk, Ł. (2019), *Zielona wyspa? Czy dżuma naprawdę ominęła Polskę Kazimierza Wielkiego?* https://hrabiatytus.pl/2019/01/21/zielona-wyspa-czy-dzuma-naprawde-ominela-polske-kazimierza-wielkiego/ [Accessed: 10.03.2022].

Kracik, J. (1991). *Pokonać czarną śmierć. Staropolskie postawy wobec zarazy.* Kraków: Wydawnictwo M.

Kracik, J. (2012). *Staropolskie postawy wobec zarazy.* Kraków: PETRUS.

Kronika Pawła Piaseckiego (1870). *Kronika Pawła Piaseckiego biskupa przemyślskiego.* Kraków.

Kuchowicz, Z. (1971). *Z badań nad stanem biologicznym społeczeństwa polskiego: od schyłku XVI do końca XVIII wieku.* Łódź – Wrocław: Zakład Narodowy im. Ossolińskich.

Lernet, J. (1817). *Rozprawa o morze.* "Roczniki Towarzystwa Przyjaciół Nauk" Vol. 11.

Lileyko, J. (1984). *Życie codzienne w Warszawie za Wazów.* Warszawa: Państwowy Instytut Wydawniczy.

McNeill, W. (1976). *Plagues and People.* New York: Anchor Books.

Mengel, D.C. (2011). A plague on Bohemia? Mapping the Black Death. *Past & Present,* 211(1).

Michalski, M. (2009). Inwazje pasożytnicze i choroby inwazyjne w przebiegu działań militarnych. In M.Z. Felsmann, J. Szarek, & M. Felsmann (Eds.), *Dawna Medycyna i Weterynaria Militarna.* Chełmno: Towarzystwo Przyjaciół Dolnej Wisły.

Mieszkowski, Ł. (2020). *Największa. Pandemia hiszpanki u progu niepodległej Polski.* Warszawa: Polityka.

Namaczyńska, S. (1937). *Kronika klęsk elementarnych w Polsce i w krajach sąsiednich w latach 1648-1696.* Lwów: Kasa im. Mianowskiego – Instytut Popierania Polskiej Twórczości Naukowej.

Naphy, W., & Spicer, A. (2004). *Czarna Śmierć.* Warszawa: PIW.

Nawrocka, M.M. (2008). Epidemie, zachowania, tradycje i odkrycia. In W. Dzieduszycki, & J. Wrzesiński (Eds.), *Epidemie, klęski, wojny.* Funeralia Lednickie – Spotkanie 10. Poznań: Wydawnictwo SNAP.

Olkowski, Z. (1968). *Epidemia cholery azjatyckiej w Prusach Wschodnich w latach 1831-1832. Komunikaty Mazursko-Warmińskie,* 4.

Pękacka-Falkowska, K. (2009). *Profilaktyka przeciwdżumowa w nowożytnym Toruniu na przykładzie działań administracyjnych i leczenia.* Toruń: Wydawnictwo Adam Marszałek.

Pękacka-Falkowska, K. (2019). *Dżuma w Toruniu w trakcie III wojny północnej.* Lublin: Towarzystwo Naukowe KUL.

Piotrowski, W. (1996). *Medycyna polska epoki kontrreformacji (1600-1764).* Jawor: Towarzystwo Miłośników Jawora.

Podgórscy B. i A. (2005), *Wielka księga demonów polskich. Leksykon i antologia demonologii ludowej.* Katowice: Wydawnictwo KOS.

Popiołek, B. (2016). Powietrzem tknięty. Zarazy i klęski żywiołowe w świadomości społecznej czasów saskich. In K. Polek, & Ł.T. Sroka (Eds.), *Epidemie w dziejach Europy. Konsekwencje społeczne, gospodarcze i kulturowe.* Kraków: Wydawnictwo Naukowe Uniwersytetu Pedagogicznego.

Prawa, przywileje i statuta miasta Krakowa (1909). Vol. 1 (1507-1586), Vol. 2 (1587-1696), Kraków: F. Piekosiński, S. Krzyżanowski.

Prucek, J. (1991). *Olomoucky morový sloup ve světle archivnich dokladů*. Okresni Archiv v Olomouci [1992 edition].

Ptaśnik, J. (1903). Powietrze w Krakowie w wieku XVI. In *Obrazki z przeszłości Krakowa*, seria 1–2, 2 vol. (88; 127 s.). Kraków: Towarzystwo Miłośników Historji i Zabytków.

Reinhardt, W. (2006). *Lebensformen Europas. Eine historische Kulturantropoligie*. München: C.H. Beck Verlag.

Rosalak, M. (2020). *Wielkie zarazy ludzkości. Jak choroby i epidemie wpływały na dzieje cywilizacji*. Warszawa: FRONDA.

Rożek, M. (2016). *Magia, Alchemia i... królewskie horoskopy*. Kraków: Petrus.

Ruffié, J., & Sournia, J.Ch. (1996). *Historia epidemii. Od dżumy do AIDS*. Warszawa: W.A.B.

Rutkowska-Płachcińska, A. (1978). Dżuma w Europie Zachodniej w XIV w. – straty demograficzne i skutki psychiczne. *Przegląd Historyczny*, 69(1).

Salmonowicz, S. (1983). Toruń wobec zarazy w XVII i XVIII wieku. *Rocznik Toruński*, 16.

Shah, S. (2020). *Epidemia. Od dżumy przez AIDS i ebolę po COVID-19*. Kraków: Znak Horyzont.

Sobków, M. (2000). *Ospa we Wrocławiu*. Wydawnictwo: Usługi Wydawnicze Ernest Dyczek.

Sokół, S. (1960). *Medycyna w Gdańsku w dobie Odrodzenia*. Wrocław-Warszawa: Zakład Narodowy im. Ossolińskich – Wydawnictwo PAN.

Srogosz, T. (1997). *Dżuma ujarzmiona? Walka z czarną śmiercią za Stanisława Augusta*. Wrocław: Wydawnictwo Arboretum.

Strong, R.P. (1920). *Typhus fever with particular reference to the Serbian epidemic*. Cambridge: Harvard University Press.

Szczęsny, W. (2020). Koronawirus nie jest pierwszy. Dlaczego epidemia dżumy w XIV wieku oszczędziła Polskę? (Interview with Dr Katarzyna Pękacka-Falkowska from the Department of History and Philosophy of Medical Sciences at the Poznań University of Medical Sciences). *Polska The Times*, 07.03.2020.

Trask, D.F. (1983). Disease in the Aftermath of War: Disaster Aid to Poland and Russia after World War I. In G.M. Foster (Ed.), *The Demands of Humanity: Army Medical Disaster Relief*. Washington, DC.

Treder, M. (2012). *Pandemie zagrożeniem XXI wieku*. Warszawa: Oficyna Wydawnicza Łośgraf.

Umiastowski, P. (1591). *Nauka o morowym powietrzu*. Kraków: Drukarnia Andrzeja Piotrkowczyka.

Urban, J. (2016). *Nasz arcybiskup. Adam Stefan Sapieha w świetle dzienników i listów Matyldy z Windisch-Graetzów Sapieżyny. Studia Sandomierskie*, 23.

Vorbeck-Lettow, M. (1968). *Skarbnica pamięci*, Wrocław: Zakład Narodowy im. Ossolińskich.

Walawender, A. (1932). *Kronika klęsk elementarnych w Polsce i w krajach sąsiednich w latach 1450–1586*. Lwów: Kasa im. J. Mianowskiego – Instytut Popierania Polskiej Twórczości Naukowe.

Walawender, A. (1957), Obrona przed zarazami w Polsce na przełomie wieków średnich. *Archiwum Historii Medycyny*, 20(1–2).

Wnęk, J. (2014). *Pandemia grypy hiszpanki (1918–1919) w świetle polskiej prasy. Archiwum Historii i Filozofii Medycyny*, 77.

Wnęk, K. (2015). Epidemia choilery w Krakowie w 1866 roku. Analiza demograficzna i przestrzenna. *Przeszłość demograficzna Polski*, 37(3).

Wójcik, D. (2006). Pallidus his equus est. Eqüs ejus, mortis imago. Wizualizacje dżumy w XVII- i XVIII-wiecznej dekoracji epitafialnej Prus Książęcych. In S. Achremczyk (Ed.), *Między barokiem a oświeceniem. Radości i troski życia codziennego*. Olsztyn: Ośrodek badań naukowych im. Wojciecha Kętrzyńskiego.

Wright, J. (2020). *Co nas (nie) zabije. Największe plagi w historii ludzkości*. Poznań: Wydawnictwo Poznańskie.

Wrzesiński, S. (2008). *Oddech śmierci. Życie codzienne podczas epidemii*. Kraków: Wydawnictwo EGIS.

Wrzesiński, S. (2011). *Epidemie w dawnej Polsce*. Warszawa: Replika.

Wyrobisz, A. (1999). Misericordia pestis tempore. Postawy i zachowania w czasie zarazy w Polsce nowożytnej (XVI-XVIII wiek). In A. Augustyniak, & U. Karpiński (Eds.), *Charitas. Miłosierdzie i opieka społeczna w ideologii, normach postępowania i praktyce społeczności wyznaniowych w Rzeczypospolitej XVI-XVIII wieku*. Warszawa: Wydawnictwo Naukowe Semper.

Złotorzycka, J. (1998). *Profesor Rudolf Weigl (1883–1957) i jego instytut. Analecta*, 7(1), 13.

Zwoliński, A. (2020). *Od powietrza ...Ludzie w czas zarazy*. Kraków: PETRUS.

# 2 Countries in Central Europe and the pandemic

*Marta Balcerek-Kosiarz*

This chapter presents the role of selected countries in Central Europe during the pandemic. On the examples of Poland, the Czech Republic, Slovakia and Hungary (V4), the scope and course of the pandemic as well as the elements of governmental strategies to combat the SARS-CoV-2 virus are presented. Based on an analysis of governmental strategies, abuses of political, corrupt and economic nature have been identified. The consequences of the pandemic are the result of a causal relationship that was directly triggered by the strategies to combat COVID-19 and indirectly triggered by the resulting abuses of power.

The chapter discusses the use of the COVID-19 pandemic as a circumstance that empowers the governing authorities of the V4 countries to violate the rights and freedoms of citizens and, on the other hand, provides justification for any action aimed at maintaining power by the current political groups. The COVID-19 pandemic exposes the ruling authorities' mechanism of appealing to higher values, such as the life or health of individuals, in order to pursue a political agenda that, in a situation of limited social activity caused by anti-COVID restrictions, can be implemented more quickly and efficiently. Hence, the presented elements of government strategies will be shown as means of exercising power. On the basis of their evaluation, abuses are pointed out, the common denominator of which is the desire of the ruling camp to maintain power. All anti-COVID measures taken are treated as political campaigning or election campaigning (Poland) in times of the pandemic crisis.

The chapter also aims to assess Poland, the Czech Republic, Slovakia and Hungary's fight against the effects of the pandemic in a time perspective covering the period from 4 March 2020 to 30 June 2021. For the purpose of this chapter, the following research questions have been formulated: Why is it important to report pandemic data to the World Health Organization (WHO) and what problems does this raise for the V4 countries? Why are there differences in information on the status of the pandemic between the data that international organisations and national governments have? Has there been misinformation of V4 citizens about the pandemic situation? Is there a causal relationship between the type of pandemic-related data

DOI: 10.4324/9781003353812-3

provided in a country and the strategic actions of those in power? What is the relationship between the central government's policy direction to date and the areas in which action has been taken? Is there a link between the government's strategy to combat COVID-19 and abuses, and (if there is) what is it? Why have the most severe social, economic and political impacts caused by the pandemic occurred in areas of abuse of power?

In this chapter, an attempt was made to verify the main hypothesis, which assumed that in Poland, the Czech Republic, Slovakia and Hungary the course of the pandemic was similar but differed in the introduced countermeasures. An auxiliary hypothesis has also been developed attempting to verify the assumption that the countries of Central Europe, apart from the problems associated with the COVID-19 pandemic, which are universal in nature, are characterised by greater susceptibility to breaking and circumventing the law in force due to the internal situation in the country.

## 2.1 The course and scope of the pandemic in Central Europe

The course and scope of the pandemic in Poland, the Czech Republic, Slovakia and Hungary has been examined to find answers to the following research questions: Why is it important to report pandemic data to WHO and what problems does this raise for the V4 countries? Why are there differences in information on pandemic status between the data that international organisations and national governments have? Has there been misinformation of V4 citizens about the pandemic situation?

Based on the number of infections and deaths caused by the SARS-CoV-2 virus, the World Health Organisation declared a coronavirus pandemic on 10 March 2020. The term "pandemic" means the spread of a new disease worldwide (Singer et al., 2021). In Poland, the Czech Republic, Slovakia and Hungary, the data reporting system is conditioned by the EU legislation and the WHO guidelines.

According to Regulation (EC) No. 1338/2008 of the European Parliament (Regulation of 16 December 2008) and of the Council of 16 December 2008 and implementing act No. 328/2011 (Act of 5 April 2011), the countries in question are obliged to report data on causes of death in accordance with the structure and scope defined in the regulation. On 20 April 2020, WHO implemented the current guidelines in this regard. According to them, a new cause of death related to the SARS-CoV-2 pandemic was introduced for statistical purposes. The guidelines take into account: cause of death (direct, secondary and underlying), co-morbidities and confirmation of SARS-CoV-2 infection (positive test result). In order to be able to code the death due to COVID-19, the World Health Organisation has created a new code U07.1 with priority in the sequence of events and a code U07.2 recommended for use in the patient's medical record when COVID-19 is suspected (probable case) until the molecular test result is available (Państwowy Zakład Higieny, 2020).

Implementation of the WHO guidelines in the Czech Republic, Slovakia and Hungary did not present difficulties as there was a consistent methodology for data collection and coding. Problems occurred in Poland, where there was no unified methodology for collecting information on the number of infected persons until 26 November 2020. The data differed depending on the entity conducting activities for statistical purposes. Eventually, the approach of the National Sanitary Inspectorate was adopted, where the number of infections corresponds to the number of persons with a positive test result. The reasons for this state of affairs resulted from:

the Polish legal order not being compatible with the WHO guidelines;
the lack of link between the crisis management system;
the data collection during the pandemic;
the multiplicity of entities collecting the same information;
the inactivity of the central authorities as regards the development of a comprehensive strategy for combating COVID-19;
the protracted implementation of procedural changes.

The obligation to enter three causes of death is implemented by all V4 countries at the national level. Thus, in Poland, the Czech Republic, Slovakia and Hungary, the physician declaring death is obliged to enter three causes of death on the death certificate: direct – the description of the disease (injury) that became the final cause of death; secondary – the condition giving rise to the direct cause of death; and underlying (primary) – the disease or circumstances of an accident, injury, poisoning that initiated the chain of disease events leading directly to death. The doctor issuing the death certificate is not entitled to code the causes; they are only obliged to describe verbally the medical conditions and other circumstances contributing to death.

According to the World Health Organisation guidelines, data on the three causes of death are collected and coded at the national level, taking into account co-morbidities. No international organisation (neither WHO nor the EU) has obliged countries to report on the three causes of death. Consequently, the extent of data reported to WHO depends on the country. Unlike Hungary, Poland, the Czech Republic and Slovakia report only one cause of death.

The lack of implementation of the WHO guidelines by Poland, the Czech Republic and Slovakia at the international level is not only due to the lack of mandatory reporting but also to the current coding process for causes of death, the main reason for this being the lack of an electronic death certificate.

The introduction of an electronic death certificate and obtaining medical information directly from healthcare units would definitely improve the reporting process. This, in turn, would make it possible to implement software for its automation (automatic coding), within which it would be possible to code all causes of death given on the certificate. This would involve fundamental legal changes to the existing regulations on medical records and the template of the death certificate, which would introduce an electronic form of this document.

Of the Visegrad countries, Hungary was the first to introduce the electronic death certificate. Work on it is not underway in the Czech Republic and Slovakia. In Poland, the software for automatic coding of causes of death has been in development by the Statistical Office in Olsztyn since 2011. It is an adaptation of the IRIS system developed for the needs of other countries by Sweden and France in cooperation with representatives of Germany, Hungary and Italy (GUS, 2021). The introduction of the same form of the electronic death certificate will ensure consistency of the information provided. This is important not only from a statistical perspective but also from a strategic one, as it enables appropriate health policy to be pursued at the central level.

Information on the course and scope of the pandemic in the V4 countries is therefore asymmetric. The asymmetry lies in the discrepancies between the data collected at national level and that reported to the World Health Organisation, leading to misinformation among citizens.

Poland, the Czech Republic and Slovakia do not provide complete data on the causes of death to the international level. Thus, there is a discrepancy between the scope of collecting and coding of mandatory data on causes of death at the national level and the scope of their reporting at the international level to WHO. The WHO's inconsistency in the use of national-level data distorts the picture of the pandemic situation within countries and causes risks of using erroneous countermeasures.

Therefore, on the basis of the data provided, it is not known whether there was a co-morbidity in addition to COVID-19 that could have been the cause of death. The extent of the data provided by Poland, the Czech Republic and Slovakia distorts the picture of the true cause of death, leading to an exaggeration of the magnitude of the incidence of the illness and falsifies the WHO's decision-making process leading to the declaration of an epidemic or pandemic.

The above analysis shows that the WHO methodology in terms of coding causes of death differs from the data submitted for analysis. And the guidelines implemented since April 2020 are unsuited to the technical capacity of the countries required to implement them. The way data are collected may not only make it difficult to identify the causes of death but also distort the assessment of the health condition of the population, which may lead to erroneous epidemiological analyses and inappropriate prevention programmes or maps of health needs.

For these reasons, the data from governmental websites dedicated to the pandemic situation in a given country are presented. Looking at the published information, there is a common scope for Poland, the Czech Republic, Slovakia and Hungary. All countries report the number of persons who have contracted, recovered or died from COVID-19. In addition, data on the number of performed antigen tests and positive and negative results are also published. Differences in the provided information are due to the countermeasures implemented by the central authorities of the countries. In the Czech Republic, for example, the data on the number of vaccinated persons are given. Depending on the country, additional information is also provided, such as the number of people hospitalised or quarantined and a breakdown by age groups that have fallen ill. It is worth noting that government websites in Poland, the Czech Republic, Slovakia and Hungary do not provide information on the pandemic situation in other countries. In order to compare the data, it is then necessary to rely on the portals of international organisations.

The data on the number of cases vary depending on where they are published. For example, divergent data are presented on portals dedicated to COVID-19 pandemic analyses, e.g., www.worldometers.info, or university research centres, e.g., John Hopkins University – Coronavirus Resource Center. Comparing the results of statistical analyses, one can indicate on the example of Slovakia the differences in the data depending on the source, e.g., according to the portal www.worldometers.info, there were (30.06.2021) 391,642 people infected in Slovakia. On the basis of the materials of the Coronavirus Resource Center, as of 30 June 2021, there are 391,609 Slovaks infected with coronavirus (*COVID-19 Dashboard, 2022*), while on the Slovak government website the number of cases since the beginning of the pandemic shows 433,008 people. The lack of uniformity of data in Slovakia distorts the picture of the situation during the pandemic, raises communication problems for central authorities and may result in inappropriate actions that are not supported by the facts (Caplanova et al., 2021).

The information presented in the Table 2.1. should be considered in relation to the population of a particular country. On the basis of the above data, the percentage of the population that fell ill, recovered and died as a result of COVID-19 will be presented. According to Eurostat, the population of the Czech Republic is 10.6 million; Hungary, 9.7 million; and Slovakia, 5.4 million. Poland, on the other hand, has a population of nearly 38 million.

In Poland, from 4 March 2020 to 30 June 2021, 2.89 million infected people were registered (about 8% of citizens). Within this group, as many as 2.65 million citizens have recovered, representing 7% of individuals nationwide. Around 72,255 people were in quarantine. In Poland, 50,088 tests for coronavirus were performed. There were 75,021 deaths, amounting to 0.2% of the Polish population (as of 30 June 2021). For comparison, in 2020, about 7% died from COVID-19 in Poland, while from cardiovascular diseases, about 40% and from cancer, about 27% (Główny Urząd Statystyczny, 2021).

In contrast, the Czechs conducted 7,965,292 tests. In relation to the population size, the largest number of people that contracted the disease was in the Czech Republic – 1.66 million (16% of the country's population), including 263,744 people over 65 years of age (about 16% of all

*Table 2.1* Data on COVID-19 in V4 countries (State until 30 April 2021)

| Data | Poland | Czech Republic | Slovakia | Hungary |
|---|---|---|---|---|
| The highest daily number of cases | 27,875 (7.11.2020) | 10,821 (22.12.2020) | 6,315 (31.12.2020) | 11,132 (20.03.2021) |
| Total number of sick people | 2.89 mln | 1.67 mln | 433,008 | 808,128 |
| Total number of people who have recovered | 2.65 mln | 1.63 mln | 378,639 | 737,000 |
| Total number of deaths | 75,021 | 30,303 | 12,510 | 29,980 |

Źródło: https://covid-19.nczisk.sk/sk; https://www.gov.pl/web/koronawirus/wykaz-zarazen-koronawirusem-sars-cov-2; https://www.worldometers.info/coronavirus/country/slovakia/; https://coronavirus.jhu.edu/region/slovakia; https://covid19.who.int/region/euro/country/hu; https://korona.gov.sk/koronavirus-na-slovensku-v-cislach/; https://onemocneni-aktualne.mzcr.cz/covid-19; https://www.vlada.cz/cz/epidemie-koronaviru/

COVID-19 patients). In the Czech Republic, in 2020, COVID-19 was recognised as an occupational disease in 13 occupations. Nurses, paramedics, teachers and mechanics, civil servants and social workers were affected the most (Tuček, 2021). Around 1,635,407 (15% of the population) recovered, while 30,303 Czechs (3%) died from the coronavirus.

In Slovakia, the number of people infected with SARS-CoV-2 amounted to 433,000 (8% of the population), 378,639 recovered (7%) and 12,510 died (2%). It is worth noting that the population of Slovakia, in principle, did not experience the negative effects of the first wave of the pandemic (by the end of August 2020, the country recorded a total of – per capita – 7 times less deaths due to COVID-19 than the Czech Republic and more than 50 times less than the average for the whole EU). In Hungary, on the other hand, the number of infected persons was 737,000 (7.5%) recovered, while 29,980 (3%) died due to the coronavirus.

In conclusion, the main problem of the course and scope of the pandemic is, on the one hand, the reporting of data by Poland, the Czech Republic and Slovakia, and on the other hand, the place of their publication. The presentation of the way statistical data are collected and the differences in their methodology at the national and international levels made it possible to identify the means of exercising power, which is the use of statistical data to build the real subjectivity of those in power to take action in pandemic conditions. On the other hand, the differences in the scale of the pandemic presented on government websites and in studies by both international organisations (WHO) and scientific institutions, e.g., John Hopkins University, resulted in misinformation of societies.

## 2.2 Government strategies for combating the pandemic

The analysis of governmental strategies for combating the pandemic aims at indicating the causal relationship between the current direction of actions of V4 governments and the measures taken by the central authorities to counteract the spread of COVID-19. The countermeasures taken correspond to the political programmes of the groups in power in the V4 countries.

For the purpose of this chapter, the mechanisms of pandemic control adopted in the countries of Central Europe are presented. Common elements in the fight against the pandemic were the introduction of lockdown, i.e. isolation of residents at home except to leave only for important life matters, a ban on meetings and mass events, the closure of borders resulting in travel restrictions and the introduction of quarantine for foreign visitors. A partial freeze on the economy and restrictions on mobility by closing schools and universities and shifting to working remotely were also implemented. It is impossible to clearly classify the lockdown tool. At the time of its introduction, it was treated as an ad hoc measure. In retrospect, however, it turns out to be an element of the strategy to fight COVID-19, when it is treated as a starting point for introducing other countermeasures.

All V4 countries have introduced governmental strategies to fight the pandemic based on the pyramid model. The idea behind this model is to cascade countermeasures against the spread of the pandemic caused by SARS-CoV-2 based on diagnosis, isolation and hospitalisation. The basis of this model is therefore a universal diagnosis, followed by isolation of patients and the introduction of isolation rooms converted from wards in hospitals. An important element of this level is the surveillance of asymptomatic patients in home isolation by primary-care physicians. The last level is the care of infected patients in hospital wards and in temporary hospitals.

The pyramid strategy in Slovakia and the Czech Republic was introduced in its original form and included a universal diagnostic campaign based on population testing for coronavirus and a vaccination campaign. The countermeasures were divided according to three groups of people: the first group included asymptomatic patients remaining in home isolation, at the second level were infected people remaining in isolation, and at the third level, people requiring hospitalisation.

Slovaks were subjected to universal diagnostics in order for the authorities to develop countermeasures (Nemec, 2021). Therefore, Slovakia was the only country that recorded successes during the first (March–June 2020) and second (July–October 2020) waves of coronavirus. During the third wave (January–March 2021), the critical situation in Slovakia escalated due to decreased social discipline, insufficient control of compliance with restrictions and a change in the government strategy.

During the first wave, Prime Minister Igor Matovič (OĽaNO) relied on the advice of a team of health experts. Since the second wave, however, in an attempt to salvage low public support, he has significantly reduced restrictions against the suggestions of epidemiologists. The development of the pandemic led to the introduction of two key elements of government strategy in November 2020. Firstly, the government authorities began to implement the innovative idea of screening the entire population over ten years of age twice with antigen tests, and secondly, they introduced a mass vaccination campaign.

The November action clearly slowed down the spread of the virus in Slovakia, but only for a limited time and in combination with a periodic tightening of restrictions. Similar actions carried out at the turn of January and February were much less effective, which the rulers explained by the spread of the British mutation of the coronavirus. This solution was widely criticised because of its short-term effects. The widespread action of testing coincided with a more important vaccination campaign for COVID-19. A change in the principle of the order of vaccinations helped reduce mortality (concerning mainly seniors) – from 8 March 2021 only the age criterion began to apply (the upper limit for the use of the AstraZeneca preparation was also raised from 55 to 70 years of age). In turn, appeals for solidarity were met with a positive response: as part of international support, Slovakia was able to count on faster delivery (as early as March) of "100,000 doses of vaccine of the Pfizer-BioNTech consortium under the EU solidarity mechanism, a temporary assistance from Romania (five doctors and eight nurses) and the provision of 200 places in intensive care units in Poland" (Dębiec, 2021b).

A hybrid pyramid model was introduced in Poland. The basis of this model is the distribution of countermeasures according to the percentages of people who have contracted COVID-19 and have clinical symptoms and patients without symptoms (order of 13 March 2020). At the first level are patients who do not have symptoms and can remain isolated at home (approximately 80–90%). At the second level are patients who do not have home conditions for isolation and are in isolation rooms. The last level includes hospitalised patients. In Poland, voluntary diagnostic was performed. The failure to test all Poles prevented a realistic assessment of the risk status and resulted in mainly ad hoc measures being taken by the central authorities (order of 26 March 2020).

During the first and second waves, the central authorities created isolation wards as an auxiliary form of care for COVID-19 patients. They were intended for people who returned to the country with a positive result without clinical symptoms or returned from abroad and had contact with sick people and, due to the lack of sanitary conditions at home, did not have the opportunity to isolate themselves from their families (Ministry of Health, 2020). The most tragic consequences of the creation of isolation wards took place in nursing homes and 24-hour care homes, where the highest number of infected people was recorded (Jędrysik & Danielewski, 2020). To counteract the spread of coronavirus in nursing homes and 24-hour care homes, PLN 38 million was allocated from the state budget and PLN 327 million from the European Social Fund (Ministry of Family, Labour and Social Policy, 2020). Relatively late in Poland, the medical personnel authorised to diagnose persons with suspected coronavirus infection was expanded. It is only since the second wave that the primary care physicians have been included in diagnosing and supervising patients treated under conditions of home isolation.

A controversial issue in Poland was, firstly, the conversion of wards in hospitals to infectious wards for patients potentially infected with coronavirus, and secondly, the conversion of entire hospitals to single-profile hospitals dedicated to patients suspected of being infected or infected with SARS-CoV-2. In the first case, there were doubts about the criteria for selecting wards which were converted to infectious wards. The prioritisation of wards resulted in those not directly related to "saving lives" being renamed infectious wards. With regard to the transformation of whole hospitals into infectious diseases hospitals, the financial issue played a key role in the form of increased resources for the care of COVID-19 patients. In Poland, 16 temporary hospitals were built (one in each voivodship). In Slovakia, on the other hand, 13 hospitals were set up in 6 regions, in Hungary 4 hospitals, and in the Czech Republic the least – only 2 hospitals.

During the first, second and third waves in Poland, the central authorities implemented support for entrepreneurs. As part of the government's "Anti-Crisis Shield" programmes, aimed at small, medium-sized and large entrepreneurs alike, the government authorities took measures to stabilise the functioning of the market and employment. It was also a challenge to provide assistance to the tourism industry, which was reflected in tourist vouchers worth PLN 914 million. As the data shows, Polish families spent only PLN 232 million making payments with tourist vouchers, which is only 25% of the total amount provided by the national authorities.

During the third wave, a vaccination campaign was launched in Poland. Firstly, medical personnel, people in nursing homes, 24-hour care homes and sanitary and epidemiological stations were vaccinated. The next stage was the introduction of a universal vaccination campaign in order to achieve herd immunity, which meant vaccinating 70–80% of all Poles. On the basis of risk assessment: exposure to infection, serious morbidity and death, socio-economic factors and transmission, citizens were divided into groups of patients having priority for vaccination (National Vaccination Programme against COVID-19, 2021).

In Hungary, the pandemic strategy differs most from the original pyramid model introduced in the Czech Republic and Slovakia. As in Poland, no screening diagnostic was carried out. The implementation of the citizen vaccination campaign was intended to underline Hungary's policy direction of the V4 countries in combating the pandemic. Hungary is a country where political countermeasures were designed to advance economic decision-making. The economy plays a key role in Viktor Orbán's hold on power. Therefore, the Hungarian government's strategy focused mainly on helping entrepreneurs. Compared to other countries, changes were introduced only after the third wave of the coronavirus. By decrees of 10 and 17 April 2021, the Hungarian government mitigated the impact of the pandemic on the national economy and labour market. The introduction of the decrees was made possible by the Hungarian government's controversial law of 30 March on epidemic prevention (more on this topic later) (Tyszka, 2020a).

> The law suspended the application of certain legal acts, banned by-elections and referendums, and increased prison sentences for violating quarantine orders and disseminating false information about COVID-19. The law came under massive criticism from the opposition, foreign media and European institutions for giving the government very strong legislative powers without parliamentary control and de facto for an unlimited period of time. The decision to revoke a state of emergency can only be taken by the government.
>
> (Tyszka, 2020b)

In summary, the presented similarities and differences in governmental strategies indicate the direction of public policies of central authorities in the sphere of combating the SARS-CoV-2 virus and allow the identification of the area that is most important from the perspective of central authorities during the pandemic. For all V4 countries, the strategy to fight the pandemic included tools from the scope of security policy (lockdown – in all four countries), health policy (screening diagnostics and vaccination of citizens – Slovakia and the Czech Republic) or economic policy (preferential business conditions for foreign capital – Hungary).

## 2.3  Irregularities and abuses of power and the pandemic

In addition to the COVID-19 pandemic problems, which are universal in nature, Central Europe countries are more prone to breaking and circumventing the existing law, because there is a higher incidence of irregularities and abuse of power associated with previous levels of socio-economic development, governments have a greater tendency to manage through restrictions due to political connotations and the impact of the pandemic is more profound than in other EU countries.

Irregularities and abuses of power were categorised into political (related to maintaining power), corruption and economic.

The largest irregularities of a political nature occurred in Poland in connection with the presidential elections scheduled for 10 May 2020. Abuses of power were associated with difficulties in conducting election campaigns caused by the introduction of a state of epidemic emergency from 14 March 2020, and then the state of epidemic from 20 March 2020. For this reason the local self-government units were not able to perform the tasks related to organisation and conduct of elections in the municipality area (drawing up and updating the voters register, issuing of certificates of eligibility to vote, provision of polling stations and operation of local electoral commissions). An important argument for the change of the election date was also the inability of election committees to perform election-related activities due to the ban on assembly and restrictions on citizens' presence in public places and movement. The response of the central authorities was the enactment of the Act of 31 March 2020 amending the Act on special solutions related to preventing, counteracting and combating COVID-19, other infectious diseases and crisis situations caused by them and other laws (Act of 31 March 2020). Under the Act, the Electoral Code in Poland was amended. As a result of the amendment, absentee voting was introduced, for which, in addition to disabled voters with a severe or moderate disability certificate, persons who were subject to compulsory quarantine, isolation or home isolation on the voting day or who were over 60 years of age on the voting day at the latest were also eligible. On 18 April 2020, the Act of 16 April 2020 on special support instruments in connection with the spread of the SARS-CoV-2 virus (Act of 16 April 2020) entered into force. Pursuant to Article 102, the provisions of the Electoral Code do not apply to the conduct of general elections for the President of the Republic of Poland during the epidemic with regard to issuing certificates on the right to vote, postal voting, voting by proxy, the determination by the State Electoral Commission of the ballot template and the Commission's ordering the printing of ballot papers. Thus, the powers of the State Election Commission to determine the template of the ballot and to order the printing of ballots, which are extremely important and indispensable for the conduct of elections, were suspended. On 5 May 2020, the State Election Commission stated that it was impossible to conduct the elections for legal and organisational reasons. Five days before the original date of the presidential elections, the legal status on the basis of which the elections were to be held was not established. On 9 May 2020, the Act of 6 April 2020 on special rules for conducting general elections for the President of the Republic of Poland ordered in 2020 (Act of 6 April 2020) entered into force. Changes to the law resulted in new elections being ordered for 28 June 2020. The elections were accompanied by numerous abuses: failure to deliver the ballot package on time, lack of notifications about the place and date of personal collection of the package at the post office and occurrence of unstamped ballots in the election package (Państwowa Komisja Wyborcza, 2020).

There were also two serious abuses of power in Poland during the second and third waves of infections. The first related to the lack of mandatory publication on 7 November 2020 of the ruling of 22 October 2020 of the Constitutional Tribunal on the unconstitutionality of the provision allowing abortion in the case of a high probability of severe and irreversible impairment of the foetus or an incurable disease threatening its life. The ruling was finally published on 27 January 2021, more than two months after the statutory deadline (Jabłoński & Rebelińska, 2021). The second abuse was the issue of removing Adam Bodnar from the position of Ombudsman after the expiry of his term of office, in a situation when his successor was not elected. The Constitutional Tribunal ruled on 15 April 2021 on this issue, stating that the provision of the Ombudsman Act allowing the Ombudsman to perform his duties after the expiry of his term of office until his successor takes office is inconsistent with the Constitution (Sobczak, 2021). The use of the Constitutional Tribunal as a tool in the political game of the ruling camp has led to a violation of the principle of a democratic state of law and the resulting guarantee of continuity of public authority bodies. As a result, the actions taken by the parliamentary majority in Poland have led to a violation of the trust of citizens in the office guarding the protection of civil rights and freedoms (Helsinki Foundation for Human Rights, 2021).

The irregularities and abuses of power of a corrupt nature occurred mainly in the Czech Republic and Poland. In the Czech Republic the most serious abuse was the case of the field hospital built on the site of the Letňany exhibition centre in Prague. The Czech government spent a total of 65 million crowns on its creation. The hospital has not been used since it was put into operation. The central authorities finally closed the hospital on 20 February 2021. The parliamentary opposition accused the government of misappropriating taxpayers' money (Prague: Temporary hospitals…, 2021). In Poland, on the other hand, during the pandemic there was the so-called mask scandal involving the purchase of 110,000 protective masks and 20,000 surgical masks for PLN 5.5 million in March 2020 without the relevant certificates from an acquaintance of the Minister of Health, Łukasz Szumowski, and his brother Marcin Szumowski. The masks did not meet any standards and proved worthless for use (Czuchnowski, 2020).

The most serious abuses and irregularities in the economic sphere took place in Hungary. During the pandemic, on 20 March 2021, Hungary adopted a law giving the Hungarian government unprecedented powers as part of its fight against the coronavirus epidemic; the Minister of Justice, Judit Varga, tabled a bill in the parliament. Under this act:

> the authorities can rule by decree, without the participation of parliament and de facto for an indefinite period of time (the decision to maintain emergency mode of ruling would be the sole responsibility of the government). The law also allows, among other things, for the suspension of certain laws and constitutional rights of citizens (including the right to protection of personal data) and includes proposals to amend the Penal Code – including a ban on holding elections and referendums during a state of emergency and the introduction of penalties of up to five years' imprisonment for breaching a quarantine order and spreading false information about the coronavirus. Under the law, the constitutionality of government action during a state of emergency is to be supervised by the Constitutional Court. Although the adoption of the law did not mean that the work of the parliament would automatically be suspended, the possibility was allowed.
>
> (Tyszka 2020a)

There were accusations that the government is moving towards establishing a permanent state of emergency with the right to rule by decree. It was indicated that actions can be taken "within the framework of the existing legal order, which allows the introduction of emergency measures" and the measures

> taken earlier by the Hungarian authorities to combat the epidemic (such as the mobilisation of 140,000 law enforcement personnel to maintain public order, or the military taking over 140 strategic companies) are not slowing down the development of the pandemic.
>
> (Tyszka 2020a)

In April 2020, the Hungarian government ranked decrees on immediate activation of funds for the purpose of the evil impact of the pandemic on the country's economy and labour market. The commentators indicated that the introduced economic solutions are controversial from the point of view of workers and small- and medium-sized enterprises. At the same time,

> the decree of 10 April 2020 on the extension of working hours is favourable to foreign companies and is part of the ongoing process of liberalisation of labour law since 2012 in the interests of large export companies. The possibilities guaranteed in 2012 to increase overtime (...) are used, for example, by the Audi Hungaria concern, which accounts for 10% of Hungary's exports and is one of the country's four largest employers. In contrast, the 2019 law, dubbed "slavery" by the opposition, was passed with the aim of creating favourable conditions for BMW's EUR 1 billion investment. Trade unions criticised the measures adopted on 10 April and demanded that the state should be the one to subsidise wages during forced shutdowns, rather than creating conditions where workers would be forced to work up to 60 hours a week to compensate the businesses.
>
> (Tyszka, 2020a)

It should be emphasised that it is also an abuse of the Hungarian government to use the fight against the pandemic as a pretext for restricting sources of funding for the opposition's activities – by using arguments related to the need for "solidarity in the joint plan to save the economy", the government introduced equal solutions such as "cutting subsidies to all political parties in half, and to take over revenues from the car ownership tax from local governments by the central budget (HUF 34 billion, i.e. approximately EUR 100 million)". In turn,

> with the decree on the creation of "special economic zones", the government is reducing the revenues of municipal governments from the tax on industry (...). Most of the tax changes implemented at the local

level not only worsen the opposition's ability to function, but may also lead to the general marginalisation of local governments.

(Tyszka, 2020b)

The abuse of power in Hungary is also evident in the vaccination campaign – the central authorities have cut short procedures to check the efficacy of products, especially Sinopharm, even though the results of third phase trials are still unknown. "In January 2021, the Hungarian Pharmaceutical Office authorised the product under pressure from the government, which accelerated its supply through a special regulation. At the same time, Hungarians did not trust these vaccines, just like part of the medical community" (Tyszka, 2021).

Irregularities and abuse of power can also be observed in the case of the launch of universal antigen testing in the Czech Republic (from 16 December 2020). This was accompanied by a simultaneous reduction in the number of testes with the method more reliable – PCR. "The much lower number of PCR tests causes speculation that the government is trying to manipulate the data" (Wasiuta 2020b).

It can be concluded from the analysis that the largest scale of fraud in the political sphere took place in Hungary. On the other hand, the most serious irregularities of a political nature occurred in Poland in connection with violation of the constitutional rules for electing the President of the Republic of Poland, failure to publish the Constitutional Court's ruling on the abortion ban and the ban on the Ombudsman from holding office until his successor is elected.

## 2.4 The social, cultural, economic and political impact of the pandemic on Central Europe

The greatest impact of the pandemic in Central Europe, from the perspective of central authorities, was the high financial costs associated with protecting public health and the anticipated economic losses of businesses, which entailed lower revenues for national budgets. From a long-term perspective, the social consequences may include a decrease in trust towards public authorities and health services, or the problem of atomisation and alienation of the society dictated by the concern for protection of one's own health. For businesses and investors, they include loss of trust in government due to uncertainty of the political and economic situation, failure to address risks in the financial markets and unclear and frequently changing legislation. The consequences of preventive measures affect both the demand and supply side. The introduced restrictions have reduced demand in sectors such as tourism, gastronomy and trade, and have led to a slowdown in manufacturing processes. Only the construction sector recorded growth during the COVID-19 pandemic. The social consequences directly determine the cultural impact associated with the closure of schools and universities and the cancellation of cultural and sporting events.

The speed of the central government response determined the magnitude of the social impact of the pandemic in public policies (Chubarova et al., 2020). Health policy changes highlighted the problem of medical staff shortages in Poland, the Czech Republic, Slovakia and Hungary, which was also present before the pandemic. A consequence of this situation was the introduction of an order from the Ministry of Health to perform only essential medical services in Slovak hospitals from the end of December 2020 to the end of January 2021. No country has prepared an effective solution to the shortage of medical staff. The ideas introduced were inefficient. For example, in Slovakia and Poland, the central authorities introduced an order for doctors employed in outpatient clinics to work in hospitals. In Slovakia, this proposal met with resistance from the medical community and the reluctance of politicians to enforce it. As a result, its implementation was abandoned. Among the consequences of insufficient staffing in Slovakia are the failure to set up temporary hospitals, the lack of contact tracing of infected persons by staff at regional sanitary units and fierce public and political criticism of screening testing for SARS-CoV-2. The COVID-19 pandemic also highlighted staff shortages and underfunding problems in the Czech health service. Among the V4 countries, the most limited access to specialist doctors occurred in the Czech Republic (Guha et al., 2021). Difficulties in performing tasks due to lack of staff also occurred in the sanitary services. Two events illustrating the situation in the Czech Republic are worth mentioning here, namely the beginning of a political debate by the Babiš government on increasing the employment of sanitary inspection staff and equalising the salaries of doctors employed there with those of medical staff in hospitals. Doctors in the Czech sanitary-epidemiological inspection service earn 60% less than those in hospitals. A similar situation occurred in Poland. For example, a doctor on a 24-hour duty in a hospital at the Warsaw National Stadium earns PLN 80,000, while a resident earns PLN 40,000. As a comparison, a day's on-call duty in a hospital is about PLN 1,000. As a result of their high salaries, doctors in Poland do not want to be on-call in hospitals.

The social impact of the pandemic on the societies of Central Europe can be mitigated through the introduction of screening testing for SARS-CoV-2. The positive impact of mass antigen testing creates a belief in the society that the pandemic can be addressed without the need for total lockdown, as well as mobilising the population, which creates a sense of community. Reports from the Slovak testing campaign have changed the pessimistic narrative related to the lack of places in hospital and the increasingly stringent restrictions being introduced. Universal antigen testing and vaccination campaigns are seen as major tools in the fight against the pandemic. The example of the Slovak tests received attention from the UK government. This was demonstrated, among other things, by the visit to Slovakia of Boris Johnson's advisers, who announced mass rapid testing on 2 November2020 before the House of Commons and the start of the two-week testing of the population of Liverpool on 6 November.

The international dimension of screening testing in Slovakia was reflected in the support of medical personnel from Austria and Hungary in the first round of the testing (Austria sent 33 military doctors and Hungary 197 people, mainly nurses, thus responding to the Slovakian request to send 50 people). The mutual assistance consolidated positive relations between these countries.

(Dębiec, 2021b)

The social impact of the actions taken by the governments of Poland, the Czech Republic, Slovakia and Hungary was also an increase in actions implementing the principle of solidarity i.e. assisting people in the group of greatest risk. The launch of a helpline for senior citizens or the support for senior citizens in their daily activities by volunteers resulted in social mobilisation to provide assistance.

Among the political effects, we can mention the consequences of the acceleration of vaccinations in Slovakia thanks to the supply of the Russian preparation Sputnik V:

Matovič's determination to contract it was influenced by a survey commissioned by the government, according to which 5.7% of Slovaks wanted to be vaccinated only with Sputnik V, and therefore its use should increase the immunity of the entire population (almost one third of citizens were willing to use this product).

(Dębiec, 2021b)

The first 200,000 doses (for 100,000 people) of the 2 million ordered arrived in Slovakia in early March 2021. The agreement with the Russians caused disputes in the ruling coalition, which led to its disintegration in April. Opponents of the purchase insist that Sputnik V is a tool of Russian hybrid warfare and is not authorised by the relevant EU agency (in the absence of a request to that effect from the Russian side), and that this could undermine Slovak confidence in the vaccination campaign. There are also doubts about other EU countries accepting the vaccination with an unauthorised preparation as a condition for free travel in the future. On the other hand, the prime minister promised to fight for the recognition of such certificates at the community level, and he refuted the accusations of the opponents of Sputnik V,

assessing them as politically motivated. He thus appealed to the pro-Russian sentiments of a large part of the society and the long-established idea of Pan-Slavism. In a situation of crisis of Slovak nationalist groups, in which similar ideas are popular, he failed not only to make up for some of the poll support lost in recent months, but also to neutralise criticism from the left-wing opposition in favour of supplying Russian preparation.

(Dębiec, 2021b)

It should be pointed out that the effects of Slovakia's widespread testing and vaccination campaign are causing Prime Minister Matovič's group to lose support in the polls, while opponents of the restrictions are gaining it.

> The latter include Deputy Prime Minister and Minister of Economy Richard Sulík (head of SaS), whom Matovič (OĽaNO) blamed for worsening the epidemic situation. While in the elections in February 2020 SaS received the support of 6.2% of voters, it currently (January 2021) garners around 13% of the vote in the polls (during this time, the percentage of OĽaNO supporters fell from 25% to 10–14%).
>
> (Dębiec, 2020b)

The political implications of the pandemic for Central Europe include, first and foremost, the centralisation of the management of the epidemic and provide a basis for the reform of the sanitary and epidemiological services, whose operation at the regional level in Poland, the Czech Republic, Slovakia or Hungary proved ineffective. The centralisation of management consisted in the establishment of governmental organisational units, e.g., the Governmental Council for Health Risks in the Czech Republic, to deal with public health risks and to coordinate the fight against the pandemic.

> The creation of the Council, headed by Prime Minister Andrej Babiš, the Minister of the Interior and the Minister of Health, was intended to prevent inconsistent decisions by the regional sanitary services. The government decided that the activities of the services should be directed by the head of the CŘT – the chief sanitary inspector. The CŘT also includes representatives of ministries, the armed forces, the police, the fire brigade and the government representative for digitization.
>
> (Wasiuta 2020a)

As a result of communication problems between the local, supralocal and central levels, the Czech authorities did not use the potential of local and regional authorities in combating the impact of the pandemic. In order to counteract the tendency to carry out in parallel two separate policies against the pandemic on the central and local levels, a four-stage territorial system of warning about the risk of infection with coronavirus – Semafor – was introduced in the Czech Republic on 3 August 2020 (Wasiuta, 2020a). Each of the stages is subordinated to a set of recommendations for citizens and a scheme of conduct for public health authorities at the district level. In the Czech Republic, alerts are issued in consultation with local authorities.

Political effects are also evident in terms of instability in governance. The COVID-19 pandemic caused chaotic political decisions (Poland), highlighted communication difficulties between coalition partners (Slovakia, the Czech Republic) and led to a loss of political support due to the introduced restrictions and vaccination campaigns (Slovakia, Hungary).

An example of linking the pandemic situation with a loss of political support as a result of a widespread vaccination campaign is the former prime minister of Slovakia. The turning point of the coalition crisis, which lasted from March 2021, was when Igor Matovič ordered 2 million Sputnik V vaccines from Russia. As a result of the coalition crisis, as many as six ministers left the government: for education and foreign affairs, and earlier for labour and health (Snephota et al., 2021). The liberal Freedom and Solidarity party (SaS) suspended their participation in the coalition, and the coalition lost its constitutional majority in the parliament (Kwiatkowska, 2021). The government crisis in Slovakia, which had lasted since the beginning of March, was resolved by an agreement among the four parties of the centre-right coalition, which resulted in the change of government. On 30 March 2021, Slovak President Zuzana Čaputová accepted the resignation of Prime Minister Igor Matovič (head of the Ordinary People and Independent Personalities party – OĽaNO) and entrusted the formation of a new government to the former deputy prime minister and finance minister, Eduard Heger. The new government included most of the ministers from Matovič's cabinet, including – a major point of contention – the head of the liberal Freedom and Solidarity party (SaS), Richard Sulík, as deputy prime minister and minister of economy. There were also changes in the positions of minister of health and minister of labour. "The core of Matovič's cabinet programme, implemented from March 2020, in which the reform of the judiciary and the fight against corruption occupied a central place, was maintained" (Dębiec, 2021c).

Similarly, as in the case of Slovakia, the impact of the vaccination campaign in Hungary can be observed. Its effects are mainly political in nature. The introduction of vaccines from China and Russia was intended to lend credibility to Hungary's long-standing strategy of "opening to the East".

In considering the economic impact of the pandemic on Central Europe, it is important to emphasise the relationship between the political agenda pursued by the ruling authorities to date and the introduced restrictions. This relationship was identified on the basis of the industries where the most severe countermeasures were taken. The country with the highest risk of economic impact is Hungary. This is a direct consequence of its liberal policy of attracting foreign investment over the years, particularly from the automotive sector.

> Since 2012, Hungary's public debt has declined from 82% to 66% of GDP and the deficit has not exceeded 2.6% of GDP during this period; economic growth in 2019 was the highest in the EU. The government has officially ruled out foreign borrowing to fight the epidemic. Sustaining good macroeconomic indicators during the pandemic is to be served, among other things, by a policy of attracting investment from large foreign companies. They account for 2–3% of all enterprises employing as much as 25% of the workforce and producing nearly half of GDP – the share of the automotive sector alone in GDP in 2017 was

22%. The largest car factories in Hungary (Audi, Mercedes, Suzuki and Opel) announced the resumption of production back in April, just after an identical decision was taken by the Volkswagen Group authorities in Germany.

(Tyszka 2021)

The economic impact of the pandemic on the Czech Republic is directly related, as in Slovakia and Poland, to international trade restrictions (Cepel et al., 2020). The higher the value of exports in the country's GDP, the higher the risk for the economy due to trade restrictions. The risk is the stagnation and uncertain outlook in the automotive industry, which in the Czech Republic accounts for 9% of GDP and 23% of exports, and Škoda Auto (VW group) is the largest private employer (each day of stopped production of this company means a loss of about PLN 200 million for the GDP). According to the forecast of the Czech branch of Raiffeisen Bank from the first quarter of 2021, if the national restrictions related to the pandemic are extended, the decrease in the Czech GDP could exceed 6.1% (Dębiec, 2020a).

The economic impact of the pandemic is also due to reduced foreign trade. The greater the share of exports in the economy of Poland, the Czech Republic, Slovakia and Hungary, the more severe are the consequences of disrupted supply chains and the associated increase in costs. This situation is particularly acute for those countries for which Germany is the most important trading partner (Poland, the Czech Republic, Slovakia).

The above analysis leads to a conclusion that the social impact of the pandemic on Central Europe is due to the internal consequences of the fight against the SARS-CoV-2 virus in each country. The greater the political and economic dependencies between the countries, the more severe the social consequences for citizens. The pandemic exposed the unstable political situation in Poland, the Czech Republic, Slovakia and Hungary, which affects the condition of the society and the pace of economic development.

## Results:

1 Disinformation of the citizens of the countries of Poland, the Czech Republic, Slovakia, Hungary caused by differences in the pandemic data presented at the natio-nal and international levels has become the main tool for exercising power in order to use the available resources by those in power, mobilise for the support of the policy pursued, focus the attention of public opinion on the number of diseases and deaths to carry out unpopular operations and cover up unfulfilled political promises.

2 The authorities of the V4 countries took measures to strengthen the belief among citizens that leadership was being properly exercised and the opposition did not have an alternative strategy for tackling the pandemic, hence the identified irregularities and abuses of power were,

according to those in power, a side effect of counteracting the pandemic aimed at saving individual lives and health.

3   As a result of the abandonment of cooperation between the V4 governments and healthcare experts, a chaos of competences and communication chaos ensued, resulting in lowered trust in the central authorities and a potential risk of losing power. The powers rescued themselves by gradually reducing restrictions during the pandemic and introducing social assistance.

4   The pandemic should have been a favourable circumstance for the integration of opposition to the ruling groups in Central European countries. In fact, the centralisation of the fight against the pandemic at central level shows that the period of the pandemic is not the right time to build the political capital of opposition groups. The recovery from the pandemic will be the time to hold those in power accountable and to propose alternative ways out, which may translate into the strengthening of the opposition and the emergence of new social movements fighting for their rights, which were marginalised during the pandemic.

## 2.5  Conclusions

Based on the analysis conducted, the main hypothesis, which states that the course of the pandemic in Poland, the Czech Republic, Slovakia and Hungary was similar, but the countermeasures differed, has been verified positively.

Among the similarities in the fight against the pandemic in the V4 countries one can point to closure of borders, restrictions on transport and movement of the population, temporary suspension of businesses in the tourism and gastronomy industries and the introduction of lockdown, a ban on cultural and sporting meetings and events, as well as the implementation of remote classes in secondary and higher education or hybrid schooling in primary education. The differences that occurred in combating the pandemic in the countries of Central Europe corresponded to countermeasures such as carrying out universal diagnostics (the Czech Republic, Slovakia), vaccination campaigns (Poland, the Czech Republic, Slovakia, Hungary) and the introduction of a state of emergency (the Czech Republic, Slovakia).

The situation within the countries determined the specific features of the pandemic. In Poland, it took the form of an umbrella syndrome, behind which the central authorities camouflaged the true purpose of their actions by introducing legal changes that violated the constitutional principles of presidential elections. In Slovakia, on the other hand, the government's crisis management policy became the main criterion for judging its efficiency and effectiveness and, as a result, led to the resignation of the prime minister. The political impact of the pandemic has led the opposition to accuse those in power of acting for political reasons by introducing restrictions. In Hungary, the government's draft laws have been criticised on the grounds of potential restrictions on freedom of speech and the risk of coming close to dictatorship. The pandemic in Hungary has also exposed the main interest group, which is foreign capital, and the measures taken have shown that the stability of internal government depends on its support, which has been reflected in measures promoting large companies and corporations.

The chapter also partially confirms the auxiliary hypothesis that, in addition to universal problems associated with the COVID-19 pandemic, countries of Central Europe are characterised by a greater susceptibility to breaking and circumventing the law when there is, on the one hand, a lack of stable central power manifesting itself in coalition crises (Slovakia) and, on the other hand, there is a single political grouping with a majority in the parliament which undertakes actions similar to authoritarian solutions (Poland). The pandemic is therefore a favourable circumstance for changes in legislation leading to abuse of power (Poland, Hungary).

The impact of the pandemic has deeper consequences in those countries where, prior to the pandemic, the level of healthcare had been inadequate, with a shortage of medical staff and medical equipment. All the internal problems of countries, occurring before the coronavirus, were highlighted and became the main focus of the fight against the pandemic – i.e. by improving the situation inside the country, an attempt was made to solve the external problem, which was the SARS-CoV-2 virus. Hence, in Poland, the Czech Republic, Slovakia and Hungary, the internal situation determined the restrictions introduced. It can be concluded that the more unstable the political, social or economic situation inside the country was, the stricter the restrictions introduced on its territory were.

## Bibliography

Caplanova, A., Sivak, R., & Szakadatova, E. (2021). Institutional trust and compliance with measures to fight COVID-19. *International Advances in Economic Research*, 27(1), 47–60.

Cepel, M., Gavurova, B., Dvorsky, J., & Belas, J. (2020). The impact of the COVID-19 crisis on the perception of business risk in the SME segment. *Journal of International Studies*, 13(3).

Chubarova, T., Maly, J., & Nemec, J. (2020). Public policy responses to the spread of COVID-19 as a potential factor determining health results: a comparative study of the Czech Republic, the Russian Federation, and the Slovak Republic. *Central European Journal of Public Policy*, 14(2).

Czech News Agency (2021). *Unused COVID-19 field hospital in Prague to be closed*. Available from: https://www.expats.cz/czech-news/article/unused-covid-19-field-hospital-in-prague-to-be-closed

Czuchnowski, W. (2020). Afera maseczkowa. Ministerstwo Zdrowia zawiadamia prokuraturę. *Gazeta Wyborcza*, 13 May 2020. Available from: https://wyborcza.pl/7,75398,25941014,afera-maseczkowa-ministerstwo-zdrowia-zawiadamia-prokurature.html

Dębiec, K. (2020a). *Czechy stopniowe łagodzenie obostrzeń*. Available from: https://www.osw.waw.pl/pl/publikacje/analizy/2020-04-08/czechy-stopniowe-lagodzenie-obostrzen

Dębiec, K. (2020b). *Powszechne testowanie na Słowacji – główne wnioski*, Ośrodek Studiów Wschodnich, 10.11. Available from: https://www.osw.waw.pl/pl/publikacje/analizy/2020-11-10/powszechne-testowanie-na-slowacji-glowne-wnioski

Dębiec, K. (2021a). *Słowacja zaostrzenie sytuacji pandemicznej i kolejna akcja testowania obywateli*, Ośrodek Studiów Wschodnich, 25.01. Available from: https://www.osw.waw.pl/pl/publikacje/analizy/2021-01-25/slowacja-zaostrzenie-sytuacji-pandemicznej-i-kolejna-akcja-testowania

Dębiec, K. (2021b). *Słowacja na skraju katastrofy zdrowotnej i kryzysu rządowego*, Ośrodek Studiów Wschodnich, 3.03. Available from: https://www.osw.waw.pl/pl/publikacje/analizy/2021-03-03/slowacja-na-skraju-katastrofy-zdrowotnej-i-kryzysu-rzadowego

Dębiec, K. (2021c). *Rząd Eduarda Hegera – ostatnia szansa słowackiej centroprawicy*, Ośrodek Studiów Wschodnich, 31.03. Available from: https://www.osw.waw.pl/pl/publikacje/analizy/2021-03-31/rzad-eduarda-hegera-ostatniaszansa-slowackiej-centroprawicy

Główny Urząd Statystyczny (Central Statistical Office) (2021). *Umieralność w 2020. Zgony według przyczyn – dane wstępne*. Available from: https://stat.gov.pl/obszary-tematyczne/ludnosc/statystyka-przyczyn-zgonow/umieralnosc-i-zgony-wedlug-przyczyn-w-2020-roku,10,1.html

Gov.pl (n.d.) *Koronawirus: informacje i ważne zalecenia*, https://www.gov.pl/web/koronawirus

Guha, A., Plzak, J., & Chovanec, M. (2021). Face to face with COVID-19: highlights of challenges encounters in various ENT practice across the Czech Republic. *European Archives of Oto-Rhino-Laryngology: Head & Neck*, 278(3), 807–812.

HFHR (2021). *Helsinki Foundation for Human Rights 2021, Oświadczenie HFPC ws. wyboru na urząd Rzecznika Praw Obywatelskiego*. Available from: https://www.hfhr.pl/oswiadczenie-hfpc-ws-wyboru-na-urzad-rzecznika-praw-obywatelskiego/

Jabłoński, M., & Rebelińska, A. (2021). *W Dzienniku Ustaw opublikowano wyrok Trybunału Konstytucyjnego w sprawie przepisów o aborcji*. Available from: https://www.pap.pl/aktualnosci/news%2C803111%2Cw-dzienniku-ustaw-opublikowano-wyrok-trybunalu-konstytucyjnego-w-sprawie

Jędrysik, M., & Danielewski, M. (2020). *W Polsce rekord zakażeń i tragedia w domach opieki*. Available from: https://oko.press/w-polsce-rekord-zakazen-i-tragedia-w-domach-opieki/

Johns Hopkins University (2022). *COVID-19 Dashboard by the Center for Systems Science and Engineering (CSSE) at Johns Hopkins University (JHU)*. Available from: https://coronavirus.jhu.edu/map.html [Accessed: 1.04.2022].

Koronavírus a Slovensko (2022a). *Koronavírus na Slovensku v číslach*. Available from: https://korona.gov.sk/koronavirus-na-slovensku-v-cislach/ [Accessed: 1.04.2022].

Koronavírus a Slovensko (2022b). *Report*. Available from: https://covid-19.nczisk.sk/sk [Accessed: 1.04.2022].

Kwiatkowska, A. (2021). *Premier Słowacji podał się do dymisji. Potajemnie zamówił 2 mln dawek szczepionki Sputnik V*. Available from: https://wyborcza.pl/7,75399,26929257,premier-slowacji-podal-sie-do-dymisji-potajemnie-zamowil-2.html

Löblová, O. (2020). Government responses to COVID-19 in the Czech Republic: February-July 2020. *Public Health Management*, 18(1), 75–79.

Ministerstvo zdravotnictví (n.d.). *Onemocnění aktuálně. Přehled aktuálních informací o nemocech v České republice.* Available from: https://onemocneni-aktualne. mzcr.cz/covid-19

Ministry of Family, Labour and Social Policy (2020). *327 mln zł z Funduszy Europejskich i budżetu państwa na wsparcie DPS w związku z pandemią*, Gov.pl, 7.04. Available from: https://www.gov.pl/web/rodzina/327-mln-zl-z-funduszy-europejskich-i-budzetu-panstwa-na-wsparcie-dps-w-zwiazku-z-pandemia

Ministry of Health, Strategy for fighting the COVID-19 pandemic. Version 3.0 (2020). Available from: https://www.gov.pl/web/zdrowie/strategia-walki-z-pandemia-covid19

National Vaccination Programme against COVID-19 (2021). Available from: https://www.gov.pl/web/szczepimysie/narodowy-program-szczepien-przeciw-covid-19

Nemec, J. (2021). Government transition in the time of the Covid-19 crisis: Slovakia case. *International Journal of Public Leadership*, 17(1), pp. 7–12.

Państwowy Zakład Higieny (2020). *Aktualizacja wytycznych dotyczących kodowania zgonów związanych z epidemią koronawirusa wywołującego COVID-19 na podstawie rekomendacji WHO z dnia 18.04.2020 r.* Available from: https://www. pzh.gov.pl/wp-content/uploads/2020/04/aktualizacja-wytycznych-do-karty-zgonu-wg-WHO-18.04.2020.pdf [Accessed: 4.04.2022].

PKW (State Election Commission) (2020). *Sprawozdanie z wyborów Prezydenta Rzeczypospolitej Polskiej zarządzonych na dzień 28 czerwca 2020.* Available from: https://pkw.gov.pl/uploaded_files/1595959102_11-1-20.pdf

*Praga: szpital tymczasowy zostanie zlikwidowany, nie przyjął ani jednego pacjenta* (2021). Rynekzdrowia.pl, 29.01. Available from: https://www.rynekzdrowia.pl/ Po-godzinach/Praga-szpitali-tymczasowy-zostanie-zlikwidowany-nie-przyjal-ani-jednego-pacjenta,218322,10.html [Accessed: 4.04.2022].

Rozporządzenie Komisji (UE) nr 328/2011 z 5 kwietnia 2011 r. w sprawie wykonania, w odniesieniu do statystyk dotyczących przyczyn zgonu, rozporządzenia Parlamentu Europejskiego i Rady (WE) nr 1338/2008 w sprawie statystyk Wspólnoty w zakresie zdrowia publicznego oraz zdrowia i bezpieczeństwa pracy, Dz.U.UE.L.90/22.

Rozporządzenie Ministra Zdrowia z 13 marca 2020a r. w sprawie ogłoszenia na obszarze Rzeczypospolitej Polskiej stanu zagrożenia epidemicznego, Dz.U. poz. 433, z późn. zm. (uchylone).

Rozporządzenie Ministra Zdrowia z 20 marca 2020b r. w sprawie ogłoszenia na obszarze Rzeczypospolitej Polskiej stanu epidemii – Dz.U. poz. 491 z późn. zm.

Rozporządzenie Ministra Zdrowia z 26 marca 2020c r. w sprawie standardu organizacyjnego opieki w izolatoriach, tekst jedn. Dz.U. 2021 poz. 965.

Rozporządzenie Parlamentu Europejskiego i Rady (WE) nr 1338/2008 z 16 grudnia 2008 r. w sprawie statystyk Wspólnoty w zakresie zdrowia publicznego oraz zdrowia i bezpieczeństwa w pracy, Dz.U.UE.L.354/70.

*Rząd częściowo zamyka hotele* (2020). Forbes, 7.11. Available from: https://www. forbes.pl/biznes/koronawirus-noclegi-w-hotelach-zmiany-od-7-listopada-2020-r/ sref28m [Accessed: 5.04.2022].

Singer, B.J., Thomson, R.N., & Bonsall, M. (2021). The effect of the definition of "pandemic" on quantitative assessments of infectious disease outbreak risk. *Nature*, 2547. Available from: https://doi.org/10.1038/s41598-021-81814-3

Snephota, M., Vlckova, J., Cizkova, K., Vachuta, J., Kolarova, H., & Klaskova, E. (2021). Acceptance of a vaccine against COVID-19 – a systematic review of surveys conducted worldwide. *Bratislavske lekarske listy*, 122(8), pp. 538–554.

Sobczak, K. (2021). *TK: Po zakończeniu kadencji RPO nie może sprawować urzędu*. Available from: https://www.prawo.pl/prawnicy-sady/kadencja-rpo-tk-debatuje-czy-przedluzenie-sprzeczne-z-konstytucja,507620.html

Tuček, M. (2021). COVID-19 in the Czech Republic 2020: probable transmission of the coronavirus SARS-CoV-2. *Central European Journal of Public Health*, 29(2), pp. 159–161.

Tyszka, F. (2020a). *Węgry: kontrowersyjny projekt specustawy w związku z pandemią Covid-19*. Available from: https://www.osw.waw.pl/pl/publikacje/analizy/2020-03-25/wegry-kontrowersyjny-projekt-specustawy-w-zwiazku-z-pandemia-covid-19

Tyszka, F. (2020b). *Węgierski sposób na walkę z gospodarczymi skutkami Covid-19*. Available from: https://www.osw.waw.pl/pl/publikacje/analizy/2020-04-22/wegierski-sposob-na-walke-z-gospodarczymi-skutkami-covid-19

Tyszka, F. (2021). *Węgry: nadzieje na szczepionki z Chin i Rosji*, Ośrodek Studiów Wschodnich, 26.02. Available from: https://www.osw.waw.pl/pl/publikacje/analizy/2021-02-26/wegry-nadzieje-na-szczepionki-z-chin-i-rosji

*Unused COVID-19 field hospital in Prague to be closed* (2021). Expats.cz, 30.01. Available from: https://www.expats.cz/czech-news/article/unused-covid-19-field-hospital-in-prague-to-be-closed

Vláda, Č.R. (n.d.). *Epidemie koronaviru*. Available from: https://www.vlada.cz/cz/epidemie-koronaviru/

Wasiuta, M. (2020a). *Covid-19 w Czechach od luzowania restrykcjo do twardego lockdownu*, Ośrodek Studiów Wschodnich, 12.08. Available from: https://www.osw.waw.pl/pl/publikacje/analizy/2020-12-23/covid-19-w-czechach-od-luzowania-restrykcji-do-twardego-lockdownu

Wasiuta, M. (2020b). *Czechy nowy system zarządzania zwalczaniem epidemii Covid-19*, Ośrodek Studiów Wschodnich, 23.12. Available from: https://www.osw.waw.pl/pl/publikacje/analizy/2020-08-12/czechy-nowy-system-zarzadzania-zwalczaniem-epidemii-covid-19

## Legal acts

Act of 31 March 2020 on amending the Act on special solutions related to preventing, counteracting and combating COVID-19, other infectious diseases and crisis situations caused by them and other laws, Journal of Laws, Item 568 as amended

Act of 6 April 2020 on the special rules for conducting general elections for the President of the Republic of Poland ordered in 2020, Journal of Laws, Item 827

Act of 16 April 2020 on special support instruments in connection with the spread of the SARS-CoV-2 virus, Journal of Laws, Item 695

Commission Regulation (EU) No. 328/2011 of 5 April 2011 implementing Regulation (EC) No. 1338/2008 of the European Parliament and of the Council on Community statistics on public health and health and safety at work, as regards statistics on causes of death

Order of the Minister of Health of 13 March 2020 on the declaration of a state of epidemic emergency on the territory of the Republic of Poland, Journal of Laws, Item 433

Order of the Minister of Health of 26 March 2020 on the organisational standard of care in isolation wards, Journal of Laws, 2020, Item 539

Regulation (EC) No 1338/2008 of the European Parliament and of the Council of 16 December 2008 on Community statistics on public health and health and safety at work


## Electronic sources

https://coronavirus.jhu.edu/region/Slovakia

https://covid-19.nczisk.sk/sk

https://covid19.who.int/region/euro/country/hu

https://www.gov.pl/web/koronawirus/wykaz-zarazen-koronawirusem-sars-cov-2

https://www.worldometers.info/coronavirus/country/slovakia/wytycznych-do-karty-zgonu-wg-WHO-18.04.2020.pdf

PZH (2020). https://www.pzh.gov.pl/wp-content/uploads/2020/04/aktualizacja-

WHO (2020a). *Health System Response Monitor Hungary.* https://www.covid19 healthsystem.org/countries/hungary/livinghit.aspx?Section=2.2%20 Workforce&Type=Chapter [Accessed: 4.04.2022].

WHO (2020b). *Health System Response Monitor Czech Republic.* https://www. covid19healthsystem.org/countries/czechrepublic/livinghit.aspx?Section= 2.1%20Physical%20infrastructure&Type=Section [Accessed: 4.04.2022].

WHO (2022). *WHO Coronavirus (COVID-19) Dashboard, Hungary.* https:// covid19.who.int/region/euro/country/hu [Accessed: 1.04.2022].

Worldometers (2022). *WORLD / COUNTRIES / SLOVAKIA.* https://www. worldometers.info/coronavirus/country/slovakia/ [Accessed: 1.04.2022].

# 3 Management of restrictions during the SARS-Cov-2 pandemic in Central European countries

*Andrzej Misiuk, Marcin Jurgilewicz, and Jozefína Drotárová*

The current COVID-19 crisis, accompanied by the desperate actions of governments trying to control the spread of the deadly virus, makes humanity aware of the ineffectiveness of the existing, proven ways of protecting against complex systemic threats and provides a unique opportunity to learn new ways of security management on a real testing ground (Michalski & Jurgilewicz, 2021; Misiuk, 2013).

Some countries, such as Switzerland and Hungary, declared a state of emergency throughout their territories as early as in mid-March 2020. Much less than the human and economic losses, however, one can observe the damage that the pandemic and the inept attempts to control it have caused in terms of human rights, fundamental rights and civil liberties. The main reason for the ineffectiveness of the security and emergency response systems in place to date in the fight against pandemics is the cross-border nature of such crisis situations. The vigorous mode of spread of the coronavirus responsible for the dynamics of the pandemic situation limits the effectiveness of the fight against the pandemic at a mature stage of its development, even though this fight comes at the cost of many sacrifices, including the surrender of some civil rights and liberties. Since emergency response in such conditions is ineffective and limited only to protecting critical internal security systems from overload and collapse by limiting the growth of disease and expanding security buffers, effective protection against pandemic threats requires strong preventive action. However, because infectious disease pandemics are, along with climate change and the resulting extreme weather events and cyber threats, among the so-called megatrends in the security environment and are globally determined, no single country can confront them "alone" without international coordination of prevention and protection efforts. These three threat areas are global in scope and do not respect national borders and legal-administrative systems, so individual states cannot defend against them on their own. Because individual states are exposed to these threats to varying degrees, the existing inequalities, far more often than reflexes of solidarity and motives to work together to combat the threats, produce a perverse temptation to strategically exploit these inequalities to build geopolitical position and advantage. Meanwhile, the fight against the ongoing pandemic is not only a purely health challenge

DOI: 10.4324/9781003353812-4

but also a testing time for the rule of law, democracy and social justice and solidarity. The coronavirus has made public opinion aware of the drastic restrictions on civil rights and freedoms and the normal mechanisms for parliamentary and citizen control of government action that can result from epidemic emergencies requiring governments and emergency teams to respond rapidly by means of regulations and decrees, without the need for parliamentary approval and without the normal process of public consultation and debate, which are a pillar of a democratic state under the rule of law based on the separation of powers. Such situations, which considerably contribute to abuses of power, can become the spawn of serious constitutional crises. In the framework of crisis response and protection of citizens from health and life threats related to the spread of coronavirus and escalation of the epidemic, state governments are forced to introduce restrictions on interpersonal contacts and the use of many goods and social facilities, inevitably interfering with the sphere of rights, freedoms and privacy of citizens (Granowska, 2020, p. 4).

Among the most common violations in this context are:

- problems with the rule of law, the temporary suspension or restriction of normal democratic standards, in particular problems and risks resulting from the use of extraordinary powers by governments and limited parliamentary oversight of the actions of executive authorities, as well as restrictions on the validity of laws relevant to the proper functioning of the public sector (e.g. on access to public information, on openness of public life, etc.);
- abrogation of certain fundamental human and civil rights guaranteed by constitutions and international conventions (e.g. the European Convention on Human Rights and Fundamental Freedoms), notably the right to life, the prohibition of torture and ill-treatment, the right to liberty, equal protection under the law, the right to a fair trial, protection from infection and access to health care, the right to respect of privacy and protection of personal data, freedom of access to information and freedom of expression, the prohibition of discrimination and the protection of victims of crime.

In most of the countries affected by the SARS-CoV-2 pandemic, extraordinary measures and severe restrictions for citizens and many business sectors are being introduced, often balancing on the edge of legality and sometimes even going beyond it. Governments in Central European countries with populist backgrounds do not make sufficient use of expert knowledge and tend to adapt the management of restrictions to the current public mood, which results in ad hoc and chaotic measures. The reality, however, is that policymakers' perceptions of the multifaceted threats posed by a pandemic situation differ significantly from those of the general public.

Restricting fundamental rights and civil liberties in the name of security has a history spanning almost two decades, as it was the terrorist attacks of

11 September 2001 that changed the way security is viewed in many areas of policy and governance, contributing not only to increased interference by state structures in many areas of life (increased controls, tighter security measures in many civilian and military spheres, changes to data and information protection laws and procedures, restrictive entry and residence permits, etc.) and the progressive erosion of civil liberties but also to a change in the role of science.[1]

The connections between the ongoing Wuhan coronavirus pandemic, governments' actions to combat the pandemic and respect for fundamental rights, human rights and civil rights and liberties present an extremely complex set of issues that pose a serious challenge to security studies. It is impossible to fully understand the uniqueness of the current situation and to assess the adequacy of the security measures introduced in the hope of bringing it under control without a thorough explanation of the complex genesis and dynamics of the development of the current situation, which has undoubtedly been the greatest humanitarian and economic crisis for humanity since the end of the Second World War. The activity of the state services responsible for security in its broadest sense is focused on two lines of action: on the one hand, the introduction and observance of restrictions (preventive actions), which are to limit the spread of the pandemic; on the other hand, taking repressive actions by limiting civil liberties and using modern technological tools for surveillance of citizens.

The scale of state activity in these two areas is quite closely related to the level of awareness of civil democracy and the tools of independent social control. The Chinese authorities could afford almost authoritarian methods of combating the pandemic, while the "ineffective" actions of the governments of the old European countries resulted from the search for more liberal methods that responded to social needs for free movement and preservation of civil liberties. The best example of this is Sweden, where until the beginning of January 2021, the strategy of the country's chief epidemiologist, responsible for the fight against COVID-19, Anders Tegnell, was to seek herd immunity to the coronavirus. It can be argued that under conditions of free movement, ease of communication and liberal values, it has been quite difficult for the EU countries to control the pandemic. On the other hand, in countries such as China, where privacy is not valued, but also in other South-East Asian countries (Thailand, Vietnam, Taiwan, South Korea), the fight against the pandemic has been more successful.

## 3.1  Restricting freedoms, human and civil rights

It is clear that the actions of governments in combating the COVID-19 pandemic have serious consequences for the fundamental rights guaranteed to every human being, including the right to life and health. The countries of Central Europe are no exception in this respect. Fundamental rights such as freedom of movement and freedom of assembly, as well as labour, business, health and education rights and the rights of asylum seekers have been particularly affected by government action. In most countries, emergency laws empower governments to impose necessary restrictions on civil rights and freedoms if required. In exercising these powers, governments have enacted legislation detailing how various situations should be handled, introducing temporary and episodic suspensions of some civil rights and liberties and specifying how those who do not comply with the new restrictions should be dealt with.[2]

However, these measures should only remain in force as long as required to prevent the spread of the disease, and their necessity, advisability and effectiveness should be regularly reviewed. Article 12 of the UN Covenant[3] obliges states to take measures that are necessary for the prevention, treatment and control of epidemics of communicable diseases. In doing so, however, states should be guided by the principles of adequacy and proportionality and limit to minimum any necessary side effects of such measures that are undesirable from the point of view of protecting human rights and civil liberties. The measures taken must be genuinely necessary from the point of view of public health protection requirements, the extent of the restrictions on the rights and freedoms must not exceed the necessary minimum and the restrictions must be as short-lived as possible. Restrictions have been introduced on many levels. Various legal solutions have been adopted in Central European countries in order to effectively fight the pandemic, which at the same time resulted in certain restrictions of civil liberties and economic life. In Poland, no decision has been made to introduce any kind of state of emergency, which is included in the list of constitutional legal and organisational solutions. Despite the fact that the conditions for enforcing a state of emergency were met, a decision was made to use the Act of 5 December 2008 on preventing and combating infections and infectious diseases in humans,[4] which allows only for specific sanitary and medical actions. According to this act, persons staying on the territory of the Republic of Poland are obliged, in particular, to undergo sanitary procedures, protective vaccinations, post-exposure prophylactic use of medicines, sanitary-epidemiological examinations, including proceedings aimed at collecting or providing material for these examinations, epidemiological surveillance, quarantine, treatment, hospitalisation, isolation, isolation in home conditions, but also to refrain from work if there is a possibility of transmitting an infection or infectious disease to other persons – if they are infected persons, persons suffering from an infectious disease or carriers, or to comply with orders and prohibitions of the bodies of the State Sanitary Inspectorate aimed at preventing and combating infections and infectious diseases. In such a situation, the possibilities of introducing administrative restrictions and limiting the freedom of movement are limited. It proves that the authorities are not aware of the scale of danger to the health and life of citizens.

In Slovakia, by contrast, the reaction of the authorities has been more adjusted to the epidemic situation. Initially, a state of emergency was introduced, and only as a result of an increase in the incidence of the disease were extraordinary measures introduced. Subsequently, provisions in the Constitutional Act were amended to allow these measures to be extended for further 40-day periods (Drotárová, 2021). Under extraordinary measures, not only can a person's inviolability and privacy be restricted, namely by forcing them to stay at home or by evacuating a specific person to a specific place, but the restriction also applies to the inviolability of a person. The amendment made it possible to impose the obligation to provide energy, road and rail care, transport, water supply and operation of sewage systems, production and supply of electricity, gas and heat, medical care, provision of social assistance, taking measures for social and legal protection of children and care, maintenance of public order or removal of existing damage, restriction of freedom of movement and residence, and restriction or prohibition of freedom of assembly. During the time of extraordinary measures being in force, an obligation was imposed on employers to check their employees to see whether they were wearing a face mask at work and to enforce COVID-19 testing. The Slovak police had the duty to monitor compliance with the relevant legislation and prohibitions, and to impose sanctions for non-compliance. The police checked if people were wearing face masks and carried out preventive police activities, which focused primarily on places with large numbers of people, such as shopping centres, sports and cultural events, discotheques, railway and bus stations, hospitals, etc. Police officers also helped to carry out checks at border crossings. Similarly, in the Czech Republic, the government introduced extraordinary measures for a period of 30 days, which was extended several times with the approval of the parliament (Chamber of Deputies). Very soon it became clear that the existing regulations did not correspond at all with the challenges posed by the COVID-19 epidemiological threat. This required a change in the emergency law to correspond with the constitutional regulations relating to states of emergency. To this end, a new Security Act was adopted to ensure coordination between the constitutional Security Council and crisis management entities. This enabled the Czech authorities to impose restrictions and limitations on movement and civil liberties. Activities in relation to preventing the spread of the virus were coordinated by the Czech Republic's Security Council, the Constitution's crisis management headquarters, the COVID-19 operational team and the Czech government. On 2 March 2020, the Czech government began taking measures to reduce the threat of cross-border traffic: flights from South Korea and northern Italy were suspended, random border controls were initiated and people returning from at-risk countries were ordered to go into quarantine. On 11 March, all primary and secondary schools and universities were closed. On 12 March, emergency measures were declared, and on 7 April they were extended until 30 April 2020. The extension of the emergency measures was repeated until 17 May. On 14 March, all restaurants and shops were closed. In mid-March, the state border was closed, and a few days later people were ordered to wear a mask or similar face covering (and cover their nose and mouth).

The reorganisation of the health system to combat the pandemic and the introduction of restrictions on access to medical services for the safety of healthcare personnel and the continuity of hospitals and healthcare facilities undermine the right to health and its protection, and result in an increased number of deaths from diseases other than SARS-CoV-2. Most countries worldwide have ratified at least one human rights agreement obliging governments to guarantee the right to health, its protection and medical assistance in life-threatening situations for everyone on their territory. International agreements and declarations oblige governments to take all necessary measures related to preventing, treating and countering the spread of diseases. In the case of a rapidly spreading epidemic, this means ensuring that all people within the territory of the state have the same access to preventive measures, goods and services. People with disabilities and those suffering from non-COVID-19 diseases must not be denied or impeded access to treatment under the pretext of pandemic restrictions. If a government recommends or requires such measures, it must first make sure that everyone in its territory has real access to them. Restrictions on social contact and freedom of movement have also been particularly severe. The introduction in most countries of restrictions on social contact, restrictions or bans on leaving one's home, minimum spatial distances and limits on number of people in public places, shops or means of transport, as well as prohibitions on visits and quotas on visitors in private places, went far beyond the civil liberties of movement hitherto enjoyed in democratic-liberal legal systems. Particularly for people with certain disabilities and people suffering from certain mental illnesses, such restrictions can have far-reaching consequences.

At the international level, the reintroduction of border controls in the Schengen area and the introduction of restrictions on cross-border movement have called into question not only the fundamental right of citizens to freedom of movement but also the right to family and its protection. The poor economic situation that prevailed in many regions of Central and Eastern Europe after the political transformations of the late 1980s and early 1990s led to mass economic emigration. Restrictions on cross-border transport (flight bans, forced isolation and quarantine of visitors from high-risk red zone countries, etc.) limited the right of millions of people working abroad to family reunification and contact with their children. The erroneous assumption by many countries that the virus has a specific nationality has had lamentable consequences. The coronavirus does not respect borders. However, due to differences in national conditions for the development of the epidemic, resulting from the susceptibility of societies to the transmission of the virus and the accuracy and effectiveness of measures taken to slow down the processes of its spread, it is possible to speak of different levels of risk of infection for citizens of different countries. The very fact of unavailability of location data of subscribers of foreign mobile phone networks changes their protective status. The introduction of restrictions must be effective when enforced by the relevant services. In the countries of Central and Eastern Europe in the first phase of the pandemic, i.e. in the spring of 2020, when there were few infections, sanitary safety checks went well, but when the statistics exceeded the threshold of several thousand infections per day, the helplessness of the state services in these countries became apparent. This exposed the lack of systemic organisational and legal solutions. In Slovakia, an exceptional operation of universal testing of citizens was carried out. The lack of clear rules for isolating infected people and for effective control of border traffic meant that, despite the high costs involved, these undertakings did not have the intended effect.

Even more than individual, personal civil liberties, restrictions have affected political rights, especially the right of assembly. In most countries, those in power decided that the fight against the pandemic required banning demonstrations, halting referendums of all kinds and even postponing elections. The judiciary also went into a minimum work mode, which limited procedural rights, led to adjournments and increased the risk of limitations. The COVID-19 crisis also negatively affected the right to information and freedom of media. A key aspect of the right to health and its protection is access to information. Every person, by virtue of his or her inalienable dignity, has the right to be informed about what danger to his or her health is posed by coronavirus infection, what actions and measures effectively prevent or reduce the risks of infection and what efforts are being made to inhibit the spread of this deadly disease. Neglecting the duty to inform torpedoes public health concerns and exposes the health of all to unlimited risks. Particularly problematic in this area are the interferences in freedom of the press and free access to information undertaken by the governments of many countries under the pretext of combating disinformation, fake news and pushing social distancing. The decision of the governments of most countries, including those in Central and Eastern Europe, to close schools and universities also infringes the constitutional right to free schooling. The introduction of distance learning and the lack of opportunities to go to school and interact with peers particularly hits pupils with the so-called migrant background, whose parents or guardians do not speak the language taught at school or do not have adequate education to help their children learn independently.

Restrictions related to trade, closure of certain industries (notably air transport, tourism, gastronomy, hospitality, sports, culture and entertainment, and many services) and restrictions on many commercial activities undermine the freedom of economic activity and the right to work. Until the outbreak of the COVID-19 pandemic, the links between health and the economy had received little attention from either science or the public. Only the ongoing pandemic has made many people realise how interdependent the two areas are. Pandemics and how to combat them have a negative impact on businesses and on workers.

The right to protection and support of health plays an important role not only in relation to the labour market. Those who are unemployed, homeless, have no permanent address or suffer from addictions are also exposed to particularly negative effects of the pandemic. Preventive measures are difficult to enforce in the case of people without permanent housing, exposing them to an increased risk of disease. The lockdown and freezing of public life have had a dramatic impact on religious freedoms and the right to worship, as the formula adopted for closing temples has restricted the organisation of services or the number of participants. In addition, the restrictions and protective measures introduced did not protect everyone equally against the risk of infection, as they could not be fully applied to people in public collective centres. Persons who are detained, arrested or serving sentences of imprisonment, as well as persons in psychiatric care facilities, hospices, social welfare homes, children's homes and youth hostels, centres for asylum seekers and repatriates and hospital patients, are exposed to an increased risk of infection and should therefore receive special protection. In all such institutions, the state must guarantee not only the possibility of full health care but also that the rules of social distance are observed.

The severity of the violations of countless fundamental, human and civil rights restricted by the actions of governments in combating the pandemic and its consequences can only be compared with martial law. Few states follow the principle of minimalism and temporal and material adequacy in their actions. The Fundamental Rights Agency's reports on the EU pandemic situation, the fight against the pandemic and its effects on civil rights and freedoms provide a critical analysis of the various actions taken by the governments of the EU Member States in the desperate fight against the deadly nanostructure, which has been ongoing since November 2019 (Fundamental Rights Report, 2019). Nevertheless, the need for decisive action in the face of an increase in new infections and high mortality rates does not entitle the violation of human rights and freedoms, as such actions are in opposition to existing international law (Convention for the Protection of Human Rights and Fundamental Freedoms of 4 November 1950). In contrast, only appropriate strategies respecting the fundamental rights of the individual can protect society in the long term from the fatal consequences of a raging epidemic. The times are extraordinary, but they do not exempt society from the obligation to make sure that human rights and humanitarian standards are still in force and respected everywhere.

## 3.2 The epidemic as a turning point in citizen surveillance

Methods of fighting the pandemic pose new, previously unknown challenges to information security, data protection and privacy. Of particular concern is the collection and processing by state authorities of "sensitive" data and information on the whereabouts, movements and contacts of citizens in order to control and contain the spread of the virus. To a lesser extent, attention is drawn to the fact that the limiting of physical contact among people and the introduction of remote working, learning and administration have shifted social life to the Internet, creating new opportunities

for network service operators, communications providers and state authorities to conduct surveillance of citizens, severely breach confidentiality,
deeply intrude into private life and conduct behavioural profiling that even
G. Orwell could not have dreamt of. Despite the significant regulatory
advances made in the last decade in the field of data security and the protection of citizens' privacy in electronic communications, the existing rules
are still underdeveloped, and the pace of legislative change and social learning processes has not kept up with the dynamics of innovation in the IT
sector. It is clear that it is not possible to fight the epidemic effectively without ongoing, high-resolution, evenly distributed monitoring of epidemic
developments throughout the country. However, not all countries are making the same effort to reconcile health protection requirements with compliance with all EU security and personal data protection standards. Such
integrated, multi-module monitoring should provide real-time information
on the health status of the population, risky contacts or behaviours (e.g.
close contact with a person who has tested positive for COVID-19 infection
after the fact or has travelled from an area of high risk of infection, etc.),
new outbreaks of the disease requiring specific actions (e.g. implementing
additional restrictions, increasing hospital capacity, increasing population
screening, directing additional forces and resources, etc.), dangerous accu-
mulations requiring special surveillance or emergency response, etc. The
prohibitive cost of repeatedly testing and confining potential carriers of the
virus in isolation facilities, as well as the reluctance of citizens to remain in
isolation or under observation, leads most governments in Central Europe
to manage home quarantine for persons who may pose an infectious risk.
The need to supervise such people's compliance with quarantine prompts
health inspectorates to use location tools, primarily mobile device logging
maps provided by mobile phone operators, as well as special applications
voluntarily installed on mobile phones that detect through Bluetooth
whether the user has been in contact with infected people. Location data
and contact information can provide important information to retrospec-
tively trace infection chains and enforce quarantines and bans on leaving
the home.

In light of questionnaire surveys conducted on representative samples of
smartphone users in England, the US, France, Germany and Italy (Milsom
et al., 2020), almost one in three respondents cite being afraid that the app
will be used for surveillance even after the outbreak has ended as the reason
for their reluctance to install it. As many companies cooperating with secret
services are involved in the production of such applications (e.g. the Israeli
company NSO Group Ltd. providing tools for movement pattern analysis
(Ackermann & Benmeleh, 2020)), such concerns do not seem exaggerated
at all. The European Union has developed Pan-European Privacy-Preserving
Proximity Tracing (PEPP-PT) standards to support member countries' initiatives by providing ready-to-use mechanisms and tools, tested for security
and functionality, as well as support for interoperability and cross-border
coverage. There are a number of international research and development

projects aimed at creating pan-European contact tracking and risk analysis applications, including DP-3T, COCOVID and EIT. Similar solutions are being introduced in individual countries, e.g. Open Coronavirus in Spain, WeTrace in Switzerland, Immuni App in Italy, NOVID20 and StoppCorona in Austria, PrivateTracer in the Netherlands.[5]

In Poland, people sent to quarantine were urged to download and install a free tracking application called "Home Quarantine".[6] The Czech Republic and Slovakia have introduced the Multi-Source Contact Tracing application. Critics of smartphone app-based tracking tools point to them not only as too high a risk of abuse but, above all, as easy to circumvent. People intending to break quarantine rules or the ban on leaving their accommodation could simply leave their smartphone at home when leaving or invoke a permitted reason for leaving the quarantine area (e.g. the need to go to the doctor). It is not possible to read the purpose of the movement from the movement data. Many countries, including those in Central and Eastern Europe, are frantically searching for a legal basis for the use of individuals' mobility and contact data in the fight against the spread of the pandemic. No country has so far had specific pandemic legislation that would uniformly regulate the powers of the state in situations of similar disasters. However, there are various special laws that extend the powers of state authorities in individual cases. These create a varied regulatory landscape consisting of different powers of the state relating to different emergency situations and enshrined in different special laws. If citizens install spyware applications knowingly and voluntarily and consent to the use of their data and information about themselves for a well-defined purpose, then there is no breach of data protection legislation on the condition that full, reliable information is provided to those giving consent about the scope, purpose and duration of the data processing. A prerequisite for legally effective consent is that citizens know who holds their data, who has access to them, how they are processed, i.e. whether personalised mobility profiles are drawn up for each individual user on the basis of the data, and whether such data are compared with the data of patients who have been diagnosed with an infection. These conditions are rarely fulfilled in practice, which makes the processing of personal data based on informed consent in emergency situations an operationally cumbersome and legally doubtful solution. The problem is that too few citizens give their consent to the collection and processing of such data for the data thus collected to be useful for an adequate identification of risky contacts with the risk of infection, as well as the procedure for obtaining such consent, which takes time. Data protection legislation also guarantees that data subjects can withdraw their consent to the collection and processing of their data at any time. In practice, however, deletion of data is not 100% effective due to the so-called curse of immortality. Data and information which has appeared in the network, even for a short while, can never be permanently deleted from it, because servers create automatic copies of the data and it is never certain whether some users have not saved this data on some media and will make it available again without the knowledge and consent of those concerned. An alternative solution would be to legally authorise the processing of data as a state right under the epidemiological protection legislation, which empowers state authorities to take the necessary measures to protect individuals and society as a whole from imminent danger. It should be critically analysed whether the use of data on the whereabouts and movements of citizens meets the conditions for such a protective measure. Also, police regulations in most countries grant law enforcement authorities the power to obtain, store and process data and information about individuals insofar as this is necessary for the performance of their statutory tasks. The question of whether such powers also apply to persons who do not pose a threat to security and order may be controversial. Certainly, preventive surveillance of the general public is not anchored in any European legal system. Determining the legally permissible scope for interfering with citizens' right to privacy in the interests of protecting their health requires a balanced assessment of individual benefits and losses, and this does not exactly speak in favour of tracking. In the elderly population, who are particularly vulnerable to severe complications of infection, the benefits of increased protection against infection would far outweigh the losses from interference with privacy, were it not for the fact that this population group has the lowest percentage of smartphone users, which does not make it any easier to obtain the necessary data or to alert them to dangers. Applications that track movements and interactions will not help protect those at risk unless population screening is intensified and waiting times for COVID-19 test results are reduced. Notwithstanding these reservations, there are sensible ways of processing data that do not breach confidentiality and data protection laws. These requirements are met, for example, by using anonymised movement and contact data in epidemiological studies conducted to better understand the ways in which the virus spreads in a given population. On the other hand, a much more important issue that requires urgent research is the impact of the transfer of social life, work, education and administrative activities to the Internet on data security and the protection of privacy of citizens. In recent years, most legal systems have introduced, as part of the fight against terrorism, hate speech or online disinformation, provisions requiring website operators to store user activity data and make such data available to state authorities (police, intelligence services, ministries or tax inspection authorities) on their request. The relocation of many social activities to the web, necessitated by the fight against the pandemic, leaves citizens trapped. Since pandemic-proven patterns of behaviour based on remote online interaction are expected to remain unchanged in many areas after the end of the pandemic, extensive research and regulatory action is needed to increase the protection of citizens from unnecessary censorship and surveillance by state authorities under the pretext of protecting the public interest, while actually serving the interests of maintaining power and fighting political opponents.

## 3.3 Crisis management in pandemic conditions

The ongoing SARS-CoV-2 pandemic has made the authorities responsible for security and the general public in many countries aware of how suddenly and violently crisis situations triggered by pandemics of severe infectious diseases with high escalation potential can push existing response systems to the brink of failure. This was particularly painfully experienced in the spring of 2020 by the populations of Lombardy and the south-western regions of Italy, and later also by the populations of Poland, the Czech Republic and Slovakia, where the sudden overloading of the hospital treatment system forced the governments to seek international assistance.

The current pandemic has confirmed the conclusions of many previous research reports on possible epidemic risk scenarios, which warned that the safety margins of most countries' health systems, configured largely to take account of normal peacetime supply needs, are inadequate for a mass outbreak of injured or seriously ill people. Under these conditions, the obvious question arises as to which ministry is responsible for all matters of health security. In most countries, the law regulating social health issues does not sufficiently take into account emergency situations with a mass occurrence of wounded or sick people. The flexible, need-based control of healthcare provision advocated by analysts has not yet been implemented in any country. The current discussion in European governmental bodies about the state of logistics facilities in crisis situations seems to be too narrow, as it does not address the increasingly likely events that may be accompanied by a mass occurrence of injured or sick people, for example, as a result of terror. The main problem is the lack of appropriate interfaces between various links of the healthcare system (commercial hospitals, crisis management and civil defence services, rescue services, fire brigades, police, etc.), which in terms of specialisation and operation, as well as legal and organisational structure, constitute different, incompatible segments of the system originally conceived as separate, independently operating services. Most European countries, including Central and Eastern Europe, have a long way to go to achieve full integration of internal security and health systems. Health security requires prevention and prophylaxis, adequate planning of preparedness, testing, evaluation and continuous exercises, as well as consistent, clear and operative legal regulations, rapid decision-making and the availability of sufficient financial resources. In no Central-Eastern European country is there permanent cross-sectoral harmonisation between the Ministry of Interior and Administration with its subordinate bodies and the complex, decentralised health service management structures. Under these conditions, it is not possible to ensure overlap and to bridge the gaps at both the state and the sub-state levels. Most treatment facilities, diagnostic laboratories and supply entities are self-reliant, and competition between them is an additional factor that makes mutual harmonisation of their activities difficult. In the event of a sudden occurrence of escalating emergencies with a large number of injured people or patients requiring medical assistance, there is a need for joint emergency planning involving central, regional and local health management authorities and all other stakeholders in the health system, continuous adaptation of the planning process to changing conditions and adequate financial resources. Emergency planning, the authorities and services involved in crisis management, civil protection and policing and the existing tried and tested procedures are geared towards dealing with "classic" large-scale damaging events, such as natural or technical disasters or terrorist attacks with large numbers of victims. The backbone of the emergency response is the health care system, whose resources in most countries are "calibrated" only for normal, everyday needs and often prove insufficient even in normal situations. To prevent further outflow of the workforce, efforts should be made to improve the financial and non-financial working conditions of medical personnel as well as to improve opportunities for training and further professional development (Jurgilewicz, 2017; Michalski & Jurgilewicz, 2021; Misiuk, 2013).

A legal basis must be created to guarantee the provision of specialist medical assistance to all persons residing on the territory, even illegal migrants, as well as to ensure the construction and maintenance of emergency reserves in case of crisis situations in terms of protective measures and equipment, the capacity of research and diagnostic laboratories, isolation facilities, etc. Maintaining adequate safety margins concerns not only intensive care places for patients in the most serious conditions but also places for patients in a medium-heavy condition requiring oxygen therapy. Even in the event of successful containment of an outbreak, the necessary reserves in the hospital care system may be exhausted. In such situations, efforts should not focus on the abstract concept of hospital beds or ventilator stations, but on an integrated concept that takes into account the specific infrastructure required and the appropriate staffing. Through appropriate funding, training, maintenance and servicing, equipment reserves must be constantly adapted to the latest state of scientific and technical knowledge. Maintaining a critical vaccine reserve as an isolated measure may not be sufficient in the case of an epidemic with high escalation potential. Security strategies based on cross-border logistics appear to be much better. The COVID-19 pandemic, as well as the situation in the supply market of hypertension medicines in the year before the pandemic, made European governments aware of the dire consequences of outsourcing the production of medicines and medical devices, resulting in the dependence of much of the world on a few distant countries. Workers' absences in China's industry and transport due to mass disease outbreaks and quarantines, combined with border closures and airline restrictions, have resulted in limits of the supply of basic protective equipment (masks, disinfectant fluids, hazmat suits, etc.) and critical shortages in almost every country in the world. Although there has not yet been extensive historical research on the relationship between the dynamics of COVID-19 spread in the early phases of the pandemic and the level of supply of essential, basic epidemiological protective equipment, it can be assumed that increasing security of supply by rebuilding production capacities in the EU countries would have significantly protected the Member States from a rapid escalation of the epidemic in the early phase of its development (Q2 2020)[7] – the key phase for its further course. Reducing the rate of virus transmission through an adequate supply of personal protective equipment would allow time to build up reserves in the system of specialist hospital care (e.g. temporary hospitals) and reduce staff losses in healthcare due to infections, deaths and quarantines. The territorial and competence boundaries of the various services involved in crisis management often vary depending on local circumstances. In order to contain an outbreak of an infectious disease in such conditions early and effectively and to minimise the number of deaths and people requiring hospitalisation, crisis planning processes must involve all relevant entities, be continuous and be combined with practical testing and exercises at the regional and local levels. A consequence of the insufficient number and intensity of practical tests and exercises carried out so far is a widespread overestimation of preparedness, capacity and sufficiency of resources. Actual crisis situations brutally verify the inadequacy of such over-optimistic self-assessments. In Poland, emergency response plans drawn up without the participation of the healthcare service are partly unrealistic, as evidenced, for example, by the assumed numbers of patients prematurely released from hospitals in order to create additional treatment buffers. Under existing conditions, buffers can only be created by cancelling planned treatments and procedures and postponing them indefinitely. Good practices proven in the current pandemic need to be scientifically analysed and evaluated, optimised and developed for similar events and situations in the future. The aim is to ensure that healthcare facilities respond to a new epidemic in early enough time, at an early stage of its development, adapt their treatment capacity to the related needs and take measures to minimise the contact between infected and "ordinary" patients. To this end, the health care financing system needs to be remodelled, as the current way of financing in most Central European countries is limited only to normal, current needs and does not allow facilities to maintain safety buffers (reserves, stocks, training, exercises, etc.) in case of sudden, escalating epidemic events. In order for decision-making processes in pandemic situations to be efficient, accurate and rational, they must be "automated" and uniform, and based on previously prepared standard procedures. It cannot be that the responsible parties in identical situations act differently each time, causing confusion and uncertainty among the population. The first thing to do is to ensure reliable, round-the-clock communication with local health administrations and local crisis management services coordinating the fight against an epidemic. In most Central European countries, due to a lack of funds, practical testing of anti-crisis systems with exercises in the event of escalating epidemic threats is abandoned, and Central European countries are no exception in this respect. Such exercises help to verify the realism of planning assumptions, identify irregularities and optimise many detailed processes both in hospitals and in the communication between them and other links of the civil defence and crisis management system, for example, various emergency services (see Robert-Koch-Institut, 2017).[8] Also, the process of analysing and evaluating the experience of past exercises is not properly carried out if exercise reports are only available to few, selected entities. Epidemic situations require extensive risk management, taking into account all areas of healthcare, civil defence and emergency response. So far, however, cooperation between health care and emergency management entities has not been very intensive either at the regional or at the local (municipal) level. The chaos in healthcare in the first months of the pandemic was due to the lack of legal regulations obliging healthcare entities to draw up emergency plans, to continuously update and improve such plans, to regularly exercise preparedness and to ensure adequate financial back-up.

In the event of an escalating outbreak of a life-threatening infectious disease, the number of intensive care units is a critical resource. Crisis management services in no country have up-to-date data on the number and type of such posts (respiratory support, Intermediate Care, Stroke Units, vital signs monitoring, neonatal intensive care posts, cardiac monitoring posts, etc.) and their occupancy. Under such conditions, there can be no efficient, agile crisis management. More aggressive influenza viruses and other infectious diseases such as COVID-19, requiring more frequent inpatient treatment or more frequent intensive care, could lead to the collapse of healthcare systems even in highly developed countries.

An escalating outbreak of a serious infectious disease threatens the functionality of all links in the medical supply chain due to the large number of people falling ill at the same time. Equipment, medicines, material supplies and production capacity cannot keep up with the increase in demand. Functional constraints at all levels make existing safety margins far from sufficient (Wurmb et al., 2017). The sudden increase in the number of patients requiring inpatient or intensive care necessitates a rapid increase in the efficiency of production and logistics processes. For this, new regulations are needed, both at the national and the international level, obliging all entities responsible for security of supply to plan for emergencies. There are international standards governing business continuity management in various crisis situations. Security margins in supply systems are only adapted to normal, everyday situations. In the event of a sudden mass number of injured people as a result of a disaster or terrorist attack, there is a need to rapidly increase operational capacity (production, supply, rescue, etc.). Preparedness for a sudden surge in the number of patients requiring medical assistance following an escalating outbreak of an infectious disease is both quantitatively and qualitatively inadequate. It is necessary to examine what material resources are required to ensure a rapid and effective increase in the capacity to supply especially patients requiring intensive care. All entities in the healthcare system – medical personnel, pharmacies, treatment and diagnostic facilities and emergency services – must be involved in the processes of emergency planning and crisis communication. It is also obvious to introduce the obligation of immediate, automatic reporting to sanitary-epidemiological services of morbidity or suspicious symptoms which may indicate infection. All available technical possibilities for immediate action should be used for this purpose. Public places such as nursing homes, prisons, etc., as well as public and non-public healthcare establishments should be included with high priority in the circulation of information. Epidemics and pandemics have disastrous consequences for the health of large groups of people and they change the conditions under which public safety systems operate. In this situation, the need for a thorough revision of existing safety management and civil protection systems and the development of new public safety strategies becomes obvious. The coronavirus pandemic has highlighted the inadequacy of many assumptions on which crisis management concepts are based and the existence of gaps in supply and weak links in logistics chains. It has raised awareness of the need to undertake extensive research and security studies in order to search for organisational solutions better suited to current megatrends (mainly accelerating technological development, increasing importance of cyberspace, climate change, environmental degradation and increased epidemic risk, and globalisation and increased migration of people, goods and capital), causing an exponential increase in the complexity of the security environment and changing the existing conditions for protective activities. Therefore, it is crucial for the success of crisis management under epidemic threats to rebuild existing scientific capacity and intensify research. The unintended real-world experiment caused by COVID-19 verifying the ability of modern security systems to face pandemics of dangerous infectious diseases provides new insights in many fields, both in overcoming biological threats and in independent issues such as the possibilities and limitations of remote working and learning or the social and economic effects of restrictions on movement or limitations on the activities of various industries. Participation in this experiment entails many cognitive and organisational benefits that could not be obtained by any other route. Above all, the pandemic provides a unique opportunity for action learning (learning by doing) on how to respond to future expected large-scale epidemic phenomena with high escalation dynamics (Hahn et al., 2020, p. 46). The first country in Europe to undertake large-scale intervention research on organisational solutions to rapidly improve healthcare system resilience and evacuation preparedness in health-related socio-economic infrastructures, and to maintain the readiness of ambulatory care infrastructures in crisis situations, is Germany. Central European countries are emerging from the turbulence caused by political transformations without the modern scientific and research infrastructure available to Western European or Scandinavian countries, which does not make it easier to face new cognitive challenges related to dynamic changes in the security environment. In view of the outlined scenarios and discussed conditions in the healthcare and crisis management system, many serious questions arise that require urgent answers. Such answers could only be provided by intensified, coordinated, large-scale, interdisciplinary research and studies on epidemic security, which could be initiated by governments under framework grant programmes similar to the one announced by the German government in 2006. It is essential to identify research needs related to the current COVID-19 pandemic and how to deal with the emergency. The following issues seem to be particularly relevant:

- how to raise public awareness of ways in which individuals can protect themselves against infection and how to change habits in interpersonal relations that favour virus transmission?
- what measures and means can be used to effectively limit the development of an epidemic on a local scale in the event of an above-average increase in the number of cases (development of new diagnostic methods and increasing the intensity of screening the population, research and development of new therapies and vaccines, closing gastronomic establishments, cinemas, schools, kindergartens and shopping facilities and services requiring close physical contact, switching to remote work, study and administration, increasing social distance by limits on the number of people who can be indoors at the same time, limiting the number of passengers on public transport, maintaining a minimum distance between people in public places, prohibiting people from travelling or leaving home without a valid reason and limiting visits, etc.)?
- what are the economic, social, societal and psychological consequences of closing places of assembly and public facilities (theatres, cinemas, restaurants, sports venues, trade fairs and exhibitions, educational institutions, universities, administrative buildings, etc.) and temporarily freezing or restricting the activities of certain industries and business sectors?

(Hahn et al., 2020, p. 41)

In order to effectively manage the risks associated with the outbreak and escalation of infectious disease epidemics, strategic thinking requiring additional scientific knowledge, honest international exchange of experiences, and new legal solutions, new planning and their better integration into the reality of the current crisis situation are needed. Raising public awareness and effective, confidence-inspiring communication play an important role. The fight against the epidemic – even though it involves severe restrictions and limitations on rights and freedoms and a painful process of learning from one's mistakes – must be properly perceived by society as a self-sacrificing, community-wide effort, the success of which requires solidarity and coordinated action by all entities. Intelligent strategies for public health and protection against pandemic are recognised by the fact that they limit undesirable social and economic side effects of restrictions to the necessary minimum. Such action, however, requires efficient interdepartmental cooperation, designing adequate safety margins for emergency situations, and rational, responsible management of the assets and resources at the disposal of health systems (human resources, competencies, equipment, information, material, time, etc.).

An extremely important role in effective crisis management under conditions of epidemic threat is played by citizens' self-help and solidary cooperation of the population with crisis services. Sudden outbreaks of pandemics strike a population accustomed to having its safety supervised on a daily basis by an organised, professional response and assistance system. However, the population has no practical experience of crises and disasters that require self-help and self-involvement. Coping with such situations requires specific cognitive and operational competences. Such elementary competencies undoubtedly include the administration of premedical first aid, the observance of basic rules of hygiene and protection against infection or home care for the sick. In order to be able to protect themselves effectively against contact with pathogens, the population must have reliable and up-to-date knowledge of the epidemic situation, hazards and risks and know and apply safety rules, individual protection measures, legal obligations and restrictions and how to behave in various crisis situations. The population should be familiar with and use all communication channels through which the services provide up-to-date information on developments, actions taken, changes and restrictions implemented, and changing specific needs for individual protection and precaution. The population must be aware that only a joint effort and following the same rules in solidarity by all can help to control the epidemic, minimise its devastating effects, shorten the duration of necessary restrictions on economic activities, rights and freedoms, and guarantee peaceful, democratic coexistence.

## 3.4 Conclusions

In view of the specific nature of pandemic threats, the increasing risk of their occurrence and the difficulty of combating them, there is an urgent need for a society-wide discussion on the revision of existing safety and health strategies and the reconfiguration of safety systems. If responsible health and security policies are not to remain mere postulates, accountability cannot simply consist of restricting individual rights and freedoms, isolating the infected and quarantining the suspected, spending billions of dollars on unreliable vaccines and ad hoc anti-crisis measures aimed only at protecting systems critical to the security and functioning of the state from a fatal overload.

In view of the desperate anti-crisis measures being taken in the current situation by those in power in most countries – measures that restrict fundamental rights, human rights and civil liberties and deeply invade privacy – a discussion needs to be held on which interventions in social and economic life are actually absolutely necessary to halt the spread of the epidemic and how to guarantee the public's protection against possible abuses of power. The complexity of the problem not only makes it a subject of biomedical research but also requires consideration in the legal sciences, especially constitutional law, as well as economic and social sciences. In most Central European countries, epidemiological protection legislation opens up a wide field of action for governments. However, because of the underdevelopment of alternative, so-called post-normal research infrastructures that enable large-scale, interventionist research projects on an interdisciplinary basis, the study base available to decision-makers is limited, so that they lack high-quality scientific information about the effectiveness of available ways to reduce transmission and spread of the virus in the population and about the legal, social, economic and political consequences of their choice and introduction. As a result, the decisions taken must be regarded as real social experiments carried out on the basis of fragmentary, situational and superficial analyses on a trial-and-error basis, without theoretically founded and methodologically reflexive forecasting of their consequences. Most governments react automatically and quite often unreflectively in the face of spikes in infection, but there are governments that try to develop different models of response depending on the scale of the threat, trying to adapt these models to local circumstances (criticality of the situation, changes in trends, rapidity of escalation, etc.). The belief that closing schools, theatres and other public places, where the abandonment of their functions is possible, helps to noticeably reduce the spread of the virus is based on American research on the Spanish flu pandemic of 1918–1920 (Garrett, 2008). At the same time, inhibiting the rate of spread of the infection clearly causes the pandemic to be prolonged over time. Due to the changes in the forms of social life that have taken place in the last hundred years, the results of historical studies on pandemics cannot be easily extrapolated to the current situation and to societies living under different natural, political, economic, social, etc., conditions. Other research approaches need to be developed to more adequately assess the effectiveness of measures and the non-health consequences of their introduction.

Given the dynamic nature of the situation, such research should be undertaken as soon as possible and aim for the most rapid, yet possibly comprehensive, wide-angle diagnoses that take into account all the relevant aspects.

## Notes

1 In the spring of 2003, the publishers of major life science journals committed themselves to self-censorship and not publishing articles containing sensitive or security-sensitive information (e.g. which could be used as instructions for building biological weapons). However, journals publishing results of biomedical research have not joined the initiative, even though such results (e.g. in immunology, vaccine development, clinical pneumology, etc.) may be useful for the development of biological weapons (Dickmann, 2012, p. 8).

2 See: Act of 5 December 2008 on preventing and combating infections and infectious diseases in humans (Journal of Laws of 2020, item 1845 as amended); Act of 2 March 2020 on specific solutions related to preventing, counteracting and combating COVID-19, other infectious diseases and crisis situations caused by them (Journal of Laws of 2020, item 1842 as amended).

3 See International Covenant on Economic, Social and Cultural Rights opened for signature in New York on 19 December 1966 (Journal of Laws of 1977, no 38, item 169 as amended).

4 Journal of Laws of 2020, item 1845 as amended.

5 See https://gdprhub.eu/index.php?title=Projects_using_personal_data_to_combat_SARS-CoV-2#Pan-European:_Framework_for_Contact_Tracing_.28PEPP-PT.29

6 The Ministry of Digitalisation's app enables faster communication with services and better care for quarantined people. It provides an alternative to costly regular police checks, absorbing forces useful for other purposes. Thanks to geolocation and image analysis, it is enough to take a selfie every day in response to a request sent by text message by the Ministry of Digitalisation to undergo a quarantine application check at the location declared in the location form. The user has 20 minutes to complete the task after receiving the text message. If he/she does not respond within this time, he/she will receive a reminder message. Failure to respond will result in the police being notified to check for quarantine violations. See https://www.gov.pl/web/uw-podlaski/aplikacja-kwarantanna-domowa.

7 https://ec.europa.eu/commission/presscorner/detail/en/ip_22_2646.

8 Even in Germany, which is known in Europe for having the highest organisational culture and adequate resources, the last large-scale anti-influenza emergency exercise was carried out in 2007 (see: BBK, 2007). New regulations, such as the National Pandemic Plan, have not yet been the subject of regional and national exercises.

## References

Ackermann, G., & Benmeleh, Y. (2020). *Israeli Spyware Firm Wants to Track Data to Stop Coronavirus Spreading*. Available from: https://www.bloomberg.com/news/articles/2020-03-17/surveillance-company-nso-supplying-data-analysis-to-stop-virus?utm_source=_link

BBK (2007). *Bundesamt für Bevölkerungsschutz und Katastrophenhilfe: Auswertungsbericht der dritten länderübergreifenden Krisenmanagementübung*. Bonn: LÜKEX.

Dickmann, P. (2012). *Biosecurity. Biomedizinisches Wissen zwischen Sicherheit und Gefährdung*. Bielefeld: transcript.

Drotárová, J. (2021). *Úlohy a činnosť zložiek Integrovaného záchranného systému SR pri riešení pandémie ochorenia COVID-19 na Slovensku*, IPE MANAGEMENT SCHOOL, Paris, Francúzsko, MPH-02/2021, Podiplomová práca, MPH – Master of Public Health.

Fundamental Rights Report (2019). *European Union Agency for Fundamental Rigts*. Luxemburg.

Garrett, T.A. (2008). Pandemic Economics: The 1918 Influenza and Its Modern-Day Implications. *Federal Reserve Bank of St. Louis Review*, March/April, 90(2), pp. 75–93. DOI: 10.20955/r.90.74-94

Granowska, J. (2020). *Przestrzeganie praw człowieka w dobie pandemii COVID-19. Stanowisko Rady Europy. Opracowanie tematyczne OT-684*. Warszawa: Kancelaria Senatu RP.

Hahn, A., Kuffer, M., Mihalic, I., Mittag, S., & Strasser, B. (2020). *Grünbuch 2020 zur Öffentlichen Sicherheit*. Berlin: Zukunftsforum Öffentliche Sicherheit.

Jurgilewicz, M. (2017). *Rola podmiotów uprawnionych do użycia lub wykorzystania środków przymusu bezpośredniego i broni palnej w ochronie bezpieczeństwa i porządku publicznego*. Siedlce: UPH Siedlce.

Michalski, K., & Jurgilewicz, M. (2021). *Konflikty technologiczne. Nowa architektura zagrożeń w epoce wielkich wyzwań.* Warszawa: Difin.

Milsom, L., Abeler, J., Altmann, S.M., Toussaert, S., Zillessen, H., & Blasone, R.P. (2020). *Survey of acceptability of app-based contact tracing in the UK, US, France, Germany and Italy.* OSF, July 21, osf.io/7vgq9

Misiuk, A. (2013). *Instytucjonalny system bezpieczeństwa wewnętrznego.* Warszawa: Difin.

Robert-Koch-Institut (2017). *Robert-Koch-Institut: Nationaler Pandemieplan. Teil I: Strukturen und Maßnahmen.* Berlin: Robert Koch-Institut.

Wurmb, T., Scholtes, K., Kolibay, F., Rechenbach, P., Vogel, U., & Kowalzik, B. (2017). Alarm- und Einsatzplanung im Krankenhaus: Vorbereitung auf Großschadenslagen. *AINS - Anästhesiologie Intensivmedizin Notfallmedizin Schmerztherapie,* 52(9), pp. 594–605. DOI: 10.1055/s-0042-120230

### Electronic sources

https://www.reuters.com/article/us-health-coronavirus-israel/israel-to-fast-track-cyber-monitoring-of-coronavirus-cases-idUSKBN2133SP.

https://www.reuters.com/article/us-health-coronavirus-israel-surveillanc/israeli-supreme-court-bans-unlimited-covid-19-mobile-phone-tracking-idUSKCN2AT279

https://www.theguardian.com/world/2020/mar/06/more-scary-than-coronavirus-south-koreas-health-alerts-expose-private-lives

https://www.thestar.com.my/business/business-news/2020/03/21/singapore-launches-contact-tracing-mobile-app-to-track-coronavirus-infections

# 4 Major challenges facing states in pandemic conditions

*Jacek Jastrzębski, Kamil Mroczka, and Kamil Liberadzki*

The main objective of this part of the study is to examine and discuss the key challenges facing the modern state in the conditions of a pandemic. The analysis includes issues related to the law-making process, healthcare policy, digitisation of state institutions and key processes carried out by entities of the system of public authority, and the establishment of principles and mechanisms of cooperation between the state and the business environment. There is no doubt that all the above-mentioned challenges are important for the efficiency and effectiveness of the state's operations in pandemic conditions. For the purposes of the conducted considerations, the following research hypothesis has been adopted: *the modern state, in relation to the pandemic of the coronavirus SARS-CoV-2 causing COVID-19 disease, faced the greatest challenges in its modern history, which it did not have to face before, because, on the one hand, there was an acceleration of law-making processes and an increase in the number of hence-resulting errors, and on the other hand, a return to the tradition of questioning official normativity, a change in healthcare policy priorities (the fight against COVID-19 – a collapse in the treatment of other diseases), an acceleration of the digitalisation of the state and its institutions leading to an increase in threats to information security, and a change in paradigms (principles) of cooperation between those in power and the business environment. The coronavirus pandemic has also affected the processes and mechanisms of functioning of the state, public decision-making and public management, moving them in large part from the analogue world to the "digital world". At this stage, it is difficult to say unequivocally whether the state has passed this test. Some of the effects of the coronavirus pandemic will only manifest themselves in a few or several years.*

## 4.1 The law-making process during the pandemic – trends and legislative effectiveness

The pandemic required (and still requires) a number of legislative actions to adapt the law and the legal system to the challenges faced by the state, citizens and businesses. Legislation undoubtedly "plays an important role in making laws and policies to address emergencies and performing oversight

DOI: 10.4324/9781003353812-5

and scrutiny of the actions, initiatives and policies of the executive" (Ginsburg & Versteeg, 2020). However, it is important to remember that there are "differences between the COVID-19 pandemic and other common crises" (Ginsburg & Versteeg, 2020), hence the specificity of the pandemic vis-à-vis previously observed disruptions in the functioning of states and economies translates into specific issues related to the legislative response to the pandemic. This response has received almost immediate attention from social scientists as well as analysts and observers of public life, which has also translated into relatively numerous publications on these issues.

The legislative response to the pandemic consisted of a number of different legislative actions, covering a very wide range of matters. It is not an easy task to present the entirety of these actions, if only for the fact that within the framework of particular normative acts there were often provisions regulating various issues, the purpose and method of regulation of which are different. Therefore, for the purposes of these considerations, an attempt has been made to systematise peri-pandemic regulations from the point of view of their nature and purpose, and not from the point of view of their location in a specific normative act.

In line with this approach, the following classification of legal regulations can be proposed:

(a) regulations concerning restrictions and limitations introduced in connection with the pandemic ("restrictive regulations");
(b) regulations conferring legislative or regulatory powers on specific bodies or entities ("authorising regulations");
(c) regulations designed to protect specific groups of entities from the impact of the pandemic or to maintain the continuity and efficiency of institutions ("protective regulations").

The division into these categories is conventional, but it may nevertheless be useful for assessing the specific issues arising in connection with the different groups of regulations. As will be pointed out, the discussion of restrictive regulation in particular focuses on different aspects than in relation to protective regulation.

Moreover, within each of the categories so identified there may be hidden regulations aimed at introducing, so to say "under the guise" of combating the pandemic or its consequences, solutions aimed at achieving other effects, in particular ad hoc political effects ("blanket regulations"). This group of regulations, however, is not distinguished as a fourth category, because this would not be methodologically correct – the criterion for its distinction lies in the fact that under the guise of actions aimed at preventing the development of the pandemic or limiting its social and economic consequences, they would in fact pursue other objectives, such as short-term political goals of groups in power, including those aimed at strengthening the executive at the expense of other authorities, or to strengthen the central government at the expense of local governments. Such a phenomenon, i.e. action "under the guise" of combating the pandemic, may concern any of the previously identified categories of regulations, so the identification of this type of regulations takes place at a different level than the identification of three groups of regulations concerning pandemics.

The above categorisation of regulations may be justified in the context of their further analysis for several reasons.

Firstly, it is worth assessing the coherence of the legislative response of individual countries to the pandemic, where this coherence will be expressed in particular by the adequacy of protective regulations to restrictive regulations. Protective regulations are a factor that is supposed to mitigate the effects of restrictive regulations, and therefore the mechanism of operation of protective regulations should in principle be adjusted to the scope and nature of restrictive regulations. For example, if restrictive regulations impose a ban or substantial restrictions on a given type of business activity, then the protective regulations should, as a rule, take this circumstance into account in an attempt to mitigate the economic and social effects of such restrictions. The coherence of the package of protective regulations and its adequacy to the needs stemming from restrictive (and possibly authorising) solutions may be an important element in the assessment of the overall legislative response to the pandemic.

Secondly, the main issues and controversies regarding assessments of the legislative response to the pandemic are different, primarily in relation to restrictive regulations on the one hand and protective regulations on the other.

In terms of restrictive regulations, issues relating to the question of the government's use or non-use of extraordinary constitutional measures to combat the pandemic, and as a basis for introducing pandemic-related restrictions, come to the fore in the discussion. In the area of protective regulations, on the other hand, criticism is conventionally directed at the effectiveness and scale of the support provided.

The above issues have also been the subject of historical and comparative legal studies (Bosek, 2021, p. 113), including – apart from Poland – the analysis of international and EU standards and the approach of selected Western European countries (Bosek, 2021, p. 123), or concerning the Visegrad Group countries (Urbanovics et al., 2020). The legal comparison shows that Poland was the only V4 country whose government did not introduce one of the extraordinary constitutional measures. It is suggested that the reason for such an approach of the Polish government was to avoid delaying the presidential elections, which could not be held during such a measure or within a certain period of time after its termination (Florczak-Wątor, 2020, p. 7; Kustra-Rogatka, 2020; Nowicka, 2020; Sadurski, 2020; Urbanovics et al., 2020; Ziółkowski, 2020). Such measures were introduced in the Czech Republic, Slovakia and Hungary. In Hungary, the introduction of an extraordinary constitutional measure was accompanied by the parliament passing – as a so-called cardinal act, adopted by a qualified two-thirds majority – of a law on protection against coronavirus, which due to its content is also referred to as the "Authorisation Act or Enabling Act" (Urbanovics et al., 2020). Note that this is a reference to the German Enabling Act (Ermächtigungsgesetz) of 23 March 1933, which, in response to the fire of the Reichstag building, granted A. Hitler's government broad authority to rule by decree, representing an important step in the consolidation of the National Socialist power.

In particular, it seems that it is the Enabling Act and the government actions taken on its basis between March and June 2020 that provide the basis for claims that the pandemic was used in Hungary to effect regime change. As D. Héjj writes – the period of the COVID-19 pandemic

> was used by the government to a large extent to strengthen its systemic position and also to bring about an imbalance of power. The reduction of the role of the parliament during the coronavirus emergency, both strictly legislative and supervisory, was countered by the efficiency of crisis management through the shortening of bureaucratic procedures.
>
> (Héjj, 2020a, 2020b)

The legislative process was used, alongside the fight against the pandemic and its consequences, to strengthen – also economically, sometimes at the expense of local government – the power of V. Orban. The regulations in this area can therefore be regarded as being in the nature of blanket regulations which, under the guise of counteracting the pandemic or its effects, in fact serve other objectives, including political objectives aimed at strengthening the central government in its relations with local government.

In the Czech Republic and Slovakia – despite the governments' use of extraordinary constitutional measures – doubts arose primarily about the constitutionality of individual restrictions and their adequacy. For example, in the Czech Republic, the ban on the presence of fathers during childbirth triggered a public debate (Koldinská, 2020), and its temperature rose after the Czech ombudsman's statement denying the nature of the right to such presence as a human or subjective right (Vikarská, 2021). The ban was eventually lifted. The practice of communicating changes in restrictions at press conferences was also questionable, with inconsistencies being signalled between the message of these conferences and the subsequent wording of the relevant regulations (Vikarská, 2021). In Slovakia, controversy was aroused by strict sanitary restrictions, e.g. prohibiting the elderly from being present in shops between 9 am and 11 am (Vikarská, 2021), which departed from the logic of solutions adopted, for example, in Poland or the Czech Republic, where certain hours – precisely intraday hours – were shopping hours for seniors, when other persons were forbidden to shop (Vikarská, 2021). A specific issue of concern in Slovakia was the approach to Roma settlements, some of which were isolated and surrounded by military sanitary cordons, which could, however, be justified by the failure of these communities to comply with the sanitary protocol and the need to protect neighbouring population groups. Restrictions, the rationality and adequacy of which have been the subject of public debate and criticism, have also occurred in Poland – an example of which is the ban on entering forests, introduced in spring 2020. Both the legal basis for such a ban (Kubicka-Żach, 2020; RPO: Entry bans…, 2021) and its rationality in the context of fighting the pandemic (Braumberger, 2020; Kośka, 2020) was questioned. Ultimately, the ban was repealed after a relatively short time of being in force.

For the purposes of the subsequent assessment of the Polish model of legislative response – in which restrictive regulations were introduced essentially on the basis of the ordinary law and regulations issued on its basis – it is, however, important to note that the use by the government, for example, in the Czech Republic, of the extraordinary constitutional measures did not eliminate issues that are present in the public debate and legal discussion also in Poland, in particular, the possible responsibility of the state for the implementation of restrictions, in the context of their legality and proportionality.[1] This may lead to a potentially important conclusion that the model of action assuming the use of an extraordinary constitutional measure does not show, from a pragmatic point of view, any significant advantages over the model implemented in Poland, which consists in the use of solutions offered by "ordinary" legislation. We will return to this issue when discussing the ongoing debate in this respect in Poland.

Changing the perspective slightly and going beyond the area of the Visegrad Group, it is worth noting that governments of Western European countries (France, Germany, Italy) – similarly to the Polish government – applied solutions based on ordinary laws (Bosek, 2021, p. 123), including legal comparative remarks on the legal regimes available in these three countries and on the judicial control of actions taken on the basis of ordinary legislation.[2]

The assessment of the action consisting in the application of solutions based on ordinary laws – without the use of an extraordinary constitutional measure – may be made on at least two levels: the legal and the pragmatic one.

The assessment conducted on the legal level must first of all refer to the question of whether in the existing situation of an epidemic threat and then epidemic, the government had a legal obligation – resulting from, for example, Article 228 in connection with Article 232 of the Constitution of the Republic of Poland – to introduce an extraordinary measure, for example, in the form of a state of natural disaster.[3]

Article 228, paragraph 1, of the Constitution provides that "[i]n situations of particular danger, if ordinary constitutional measures are inadequate, any (…) appropriate extraordinary measures may be introduced". The provision thus establishes two prerequisites (a situation of particular danger and the inadequate character of ordinary constitutional measures), the combined occurrence of which makes it possible to introduce an appropriate extraordinary measure. These general prerequisites concerning all extraordinary measures are specified with regard to particular ones in the provisions concerning them, i.e. with regard to, for example, the state of a natural disaster – in Article 232 of the Constitution of the Republic of Poland (Steinborn, 2016). The principles of exceptionality and subsidiarity of extraordinary measures follow from them, which should constitute the *ultima ratio*, applicable only in cases where other measures cannot be sufficient (Steinborn, 2016).

Such an approach to the prerequisites for the introduction of extraordinary measures corresponds to the discretionary nature of the decision to introduce an extraordinary measure, which arises semantically from Article 228 of the Polish Constitution. The Constitution explicitly states that such a measure "may be introduced", although grammatically a wording stating, for example, that a specific extraordinary measure "shall be introduced" in the event of the occurrence of certain premises would be admissible (Florczak-Wątor, 2020, pp. 8–9). The issue is important because it raises doubts in more recent literature, where some authors point to the violation of the constitutional obligation to introduce extraordinary measures as the basis for the construction of unlawfulness of state actions in the context of its liability for damages resulting from the introduction of restrictive regulations (Florczak-Wątor, 2020, pp. 8–9; Pecyna, 2020, p. 28). Such a view is based on the statement that the public-law nature of Article 228(1) of the Constitution and the need to interpret it taking into account the entirety of the constitutional norms (in particular Article 68(4) of the Polish Constitution) argue in favour of interpreting the provision of Article 228(1) of the Polish Constitution as containing in fact the norm imposing on the addressee the obligation to introduce an appropriate extraordinary measure in the event of the occurrence of constitutional premises (Florczak-Wątor, 2020, p. 9; Kardas, 2020, p. 10), which are further specified in ordinary laws.

The concept assuming that the bodies authorised to introduce extraordinary measures are bound by a legal obligation to do so is not appropriate for several reasons. First and foremost, it is connected with the responsibility of these bodies – particularly the Council of Ministers – to assess the occurrence of the prerequisites for the introduction of extraordinary measures. The necessary prerequisite for the introduction of such a measure is the determination that "ordinary constitutional means are insufficient" (Article 228(1) of the Polish Constitution). The burden of making this assessment and the responsibility for it rests with the body authorised to take the decision to introduce extraordinary measures – i.e., in the first place, the Council of Ministers (Bosek, 2021, p. 138).

Therefore, we believe that one should agree with the position expressed by the Supreme Court in its decision of 28 July 2020 (Bosek, 2021, p. 139; Wyrok SN I NSW 2849/20, 2020, LEX No. 3043973), in which the Supreme Court stated that

> the Council of Ministers was not obliged to introduce a state of natural disaster in response to the COVID-19 epidemic, in a situation where

there was a possibility of introducing a state of epidemic emergency and a state of epidemic, as provided for in Article 46 of the Act of 5 December 2008 on preventing and combating infections and infectious diseases in humans (Journal of Laws of 2019, item 1239 as amended). The decision to introduce an extraordinary measure, due to the generality of the prerequisites for its introduction, belongs to the sphere of administrative discretion of state authorities, which means that it is up to them to assess whether these prerequisites have been fulfilled in a specific situation – e.g. the outbreak of an epidemic.

Turning to the assessment made on a pragmatic level, one must also take into account the factual circumstances existing at the time of taking the decision on whether or not to impose extraordinary measures. In the spring of 2020, there was considerable uncertainty as to further developments in the pandemic situation, in particular as to the potential escalation of the pandemic, which could translate into a significant increase in the number of infections, hospitalisations and deaths. Against this background, it was rational to gradate the legal measures used and to avoid the most far-reaching measures in a situation where the circumstances underlying the application of such measures are expected to escalate. For this reason, we believe that great caution should be exercised when making *post-factum* assessments of past decisions, on the basis of limited information and taking into account the various possible – including extremely negative – developments.

An important contribution to the evaluation of the epidemic response model adopted in Poland in the context of restrictive regulations is also provided by comparative studies that indicate, on the one hand, a similar model of legal response to the epidemic in selected countries (Bosek, 2021, p. 123), and on the other hand, practical consequences in the form of the emergence of compensation claims related to the introduction of restrictions also in those jurisdictions where, unlike in Poland, the decision was made to make use of extraordinary constitutional measures (e.g. in the Czech Republic and Hungary). This shows, on the one hand, that the Polish legislative model of responding to the epidemic – which does not assume the use of constitutional grounds for introducing extraordinary measures – is not isolated in Europe (although it was isolated within the V4), and on the other hand, that a legislative response based on constitutional grounds for introducing extraordinary measures does not prevent the phenomena consisting in contesting the introduced restrictions, as well as attempts to derive compensation claims towards the state from them.

This should not, of course, limit the process of drawing *de lege ferenda* conclusions on the basis of the experience of the epidemic. In this context it is pointed out, in particular, that reality has negatively verified the usefulness of distinguishing two states in the Act on communicable diseases – i.e. the state of epidemic emergency (Article 2(23) of the Act) and the state of epidemic (Article 2(22) of the Act). Hence, it is proposed to replace both hitherto differentiated states with one, indicating that the state of epidemic would be sufficient (Bosek, 2021, p. 134).

Summing up the Polish model of legislative response to the pandemic, it is worth noting that restrictive regulations – which resulted in particular in limitations on conducting a specific type of business activity – were accompanied by protective regulations, minimising the negative social and economic effects of the introduced restrictions. The range of protective regulations was broad and included aspects related to the use of government aid programmes, but also solutions aimed at making the existing legal framework more flexible in order to enable better overcoming of epidemic difficulties. This leads to the assessment that, at a macro level, the legislative response appears to have been comprehensive.

One should bear in mind that, under conditions of unprecedented time pressure and limited information surrounding the initial phase of the epidemic, legislators are entitled to make mistakes when drafting regulations, which may lead to regulatory inconsistencies in matters of detail. This is a natural and unavoidable consequence of such difficult conditions of the law-making process. It is also worth noting that the addressees of the law showed – especially in the initial period of the pandemic – a certain understanding of the imperfections of the legislation created under time pressure, which, however, became weaker as the subsequent months of the pandemic passed (Biga, 2020). Another issue is the legislative technique used, which due to the specific mode of work on the bills (this seems to have been particularly true of Shield 1.0) took on a form which was difficult for the public to understand, partly also due to the intention to include in a single piece of legislation regulations relating to a broad spectrum of social relations and involved amendments to many provisions of other laws.

This is in part a consequence of the barriers and difficulties faced by any legislator in drawing up regulations intended to respond to a pandemic. In addition to the already mentioned time pressure, one should also point out the significant uncertainty regarding further development of the epidemic situation and – which is particularly important – the time horizon of its duration. This is because it is completely different to design episodic solutions if the expected time horizon of their application is counted in weeks, and not when it comes to months or years. An example in this respect may be, for example, the approach of legislators to the running of time limits in proceedings, which should be resolved with certain assumptions as to the expected duration of the suspension.

In Poland, as in other countries, there was – and still is – a discussion concerning legal, and in particular constitutional, conditions for undertaking specific actions related to counteracting the pandemic or its effects. It concerns primarily two threads: the adequacy of legal tools (instruments provided for in acts of constitutional rank versus instruments provided for in ordinary legislation) and the compatibility with acts of constitutional rank of particular restrictions on personal freedom (e.g. the obligation to wear masks, restrictions on the freedom of assembly, restrictions on the availability of services for non-vaccinated persons).[4]

The background to this discussion is, in our opinion, immanently characteristic of all emergency situations and the strengthening of the position of the executive in relation to the other branches of government (exemplified by the wider use of orders in legislation, as well as the strengthening of the central power in relation to local authorities). These processes are somewhat natural and, from a management point of view, conducive to a more efficient fight against a pandemic. However, they also inevitably lead to the inclusion of political motives in the scope of discussion, so that the discussion takes on a political rather than a legal or managerial dimension. Opposition formations, especially those with an advantage over ruling groupings in local centres, will naturally raise doubts about the excessive strengthening of the executive and central power. The question here, however, should be whether this strengthening does indeed go beyond the objective of combating the pandemic or its effects – in fact, going towards other political goals. An analogous question should be formulated with regard to restrictions on personal freedoms.

A natural feature of periods during which societies experience disturbing phenomena threatening their functioning and requiring the launch of accelerated legislation constituting the state's response aimed at launching protective processes is the temptation to take advantage of systemic opportunities to "sneak in" solutions aimed at achieving particular political goals, for example, those related to the state taking over entities conducting economic activity, or administratively depriving local governments of revenues. Obviously, such solutions raise legal doubts and should be evaluated negatively. A particularly controversial issue in Poland has been a ban on assembly (RPO entry bans, 2021), with the key context being the Constitutional Tribunal's judgement of 22 October 2020 on the grounds for the permissibility of abortion. The social importance and sensitivity of the issues decided by the Constitutional Tribunal meant that a natural effect of the ruling was the need for a wide range of citizens to manifest their views and outrage – which in turn was confronted with a ban on assembly justified by the pandemic reasons. While the assembly ban itself may be considered rationally justified by the need to prevent the spread of the virus, in the context of the Constitutional Tribunal's judgement it was perceived as an instrument restricting the possibility to demonstrate views and dissatisfaction with the judgement of an exceptionally sensitive case.

The scale of the pandemic – as repetitively mentioned – took policy makers by surprise. The lack of data and realistic forecasts of how the situation would develop did not fail to affect the legislative process. Proposed and implemented legal changes often failed to keep pace with developments, resulting in public dissatisfaction and questioning of the V4 governments' activities. A general fatigue with the need for social isolation and adherence to strict prohibitions is also not insignificant for the perception and evaluation of successive restrictive regulations. In the social dimension, we are dealing with the phenomenon of aversion to the state and its institutions. It is also worth noting that existing legal regulations on the state of pandemic emergencies vary across the EU. This causes problems related to effective management in situations of pandemic threat. Perhaps the EU legislator should initiate legislative action to bring order to this area. This is particularly important in the context of the coherence, efficiency and effectiveness of the actions of individual Member States. Issues of far less importance for the functioning of societies, states and the economy than the model of the legislative response to a pandemic threat are regulated at the EU level.

## 4.2  Problems in the implementation of healthcare policies

At the beginning of this discussion, reference to Lalonde's concept of health areas will be made. Lalonde stressed that "health is the result of factors related to genetic inheritance, environment, lifestyle and medical care. The promotion of healthy lifestyle can improve health and reduce the need for medical care" (Lalonde, 1974). This model assumes the following groups of factors influencing the health status of the population, the so-called health areas: "the biology and genetics area, the behaviour and lifestyle area, the environmental area (economic, social, cultural and physical factors) and the organisation of the healthcare system area" (Wysocki & Miller, 2003, p. 506). The healthcare policy, or in shorter terms, the health policy, is defined in the doctrine as "a section of activity of public authorities at various levels, the object of which is protection of health" (Białynicki-Birula, 2013). In this context, health protection is understood as "an organised activity for the health of citizens, hence health policy can be called as a set of activities undertaken by public authorities in the field of population health" (Białynicki-Birula, 2013).

Health policy has become a key public policy in the V4 countries in 2020. The governments of these countries decided to increase spending on healthcare policy, to recruit medical staff and to introduce legislative solutions restricting, among other things, the circulation of certain medical materials necessary to fight the pandemic. Undoubtedly, intervention in such a specific matter as healthcare policy is burdened with a significant risk of failure (Nowak & Zybała, 2020, p. 21).

An additional problem was the sharp political dispute between those in power and the opposition, society and business, and the lack of consensus on key issues relating to the health security of the citizens of the V4 countries. One could risk saying that there was no horizontal strategy to fight the pandemic, and actions were taken on the basis of fragmentary data and in response to current problems rather than long-term goals. This problem affected most countries in the world, as political leaders failed to learn the right lessons from previous health crises. An extensive analysis of the omissions of states and international organisations has been carried out by Deborah MacKenzie and will therefore not be cited. However, one has to agree with the statement that "the world was not ready for COVID-19 and is generally not ready for any pandemic to break out" (MacKenzie, 2020, p. 169). Ab Osterhaus speaks in a similar and alarmist tone. He believes that "despite all the 'alarmist' calls of the past for better pandemic preparedness we only start preparing when the house is on fire" (MacKenzie, 2020, p. 169). Also in the V4 countries, large-scale activities have started when "the house was already on fire".

The above statements are covered by reports from international organisations specialising in healthcare policy. The Global Health Security Alliance's 2019 report states explicitly that "the GHS Index analysis finds no country is fully prepared for epidemics or pandemics" (GHS Index, 2019, p. 9). It goes on to highlight that because infectious diseases know no borders, all countries must prioritise and exercise the capabilities required to prevent, detect and rapidly respond to public health emergencies (GHS Index, 2019, p. 5). The V4 countries, according to the cited report, occupy distant places in the ranking: (1) Poland – 55.4 Index Score and 32nd place out of 195 analysed countries, (2) Hungary – 54.0 Index Score and 35th place, (3) Czech Republic – 52.0 Index Score and 42nd place, and (4) Slovakia – 47.9 Index Score and 52nd place. The results obtained by the remaining countries are not encouraging either. Less than 20% of countries scored above 80 Index Score in the area of detection and reporting, and less than 5% received top marks in the context of the criteria of rapid response and mitigation (MacKenzie, 2020, p. 184).

The most important health policy task during the coronavirus pandemic is to ensure an adequate level of health protection for all citizens. This requires both appropriate diagnostic measures (testing) and accessibility to health services. Importantly, accessibility must go hand in hand with affordability and trust in the system. It is obvious – albeit important – to say that the virus does not recognise borders. Wealth status is irrelevant, although the higher the economic status of a society, the greater the chances of successfully combating a pandemic.

On the basis of experience to date and an analysis of the data available as of June 2021, it can be concluded that the V4 has been painfully affected by the coronavirus outbreak. In the European Union, three of the four countries with the highest number of COVID deaths per million inhabitants are Hungary (over 3,000 deaths), the Czech Republic (over 2,800 deaths) and Slovakia (over 2,200 deaths). Poland is slightly better, ranking 9th from the end (over 1,950 deaths). The reasons for this situation are not obvious and unambiguous, if only because all other V4 countries spend a higher per cent of GDP on health policy than Poland, yet they are all well below the EU average (Current healthcare expenditure relative to GDP, 2018). Here, the first important conclusion emerges, which is that the lower economic development of the V4 countries combined with lower health policy spending has affected the effectiveness and efficiency of the fight against the pandemic. The V4 countries were, at various times during the pandemic, on the brink of the health system's endurance. Infrastructure which has nothing to do with medicine on a day-to-day basis was used to fight the pandemic. In

Poland, for example, the National Stadium and other exhibition and commercial venues were adopted to set up temporary hospitals.

The analysis related to the problems in the implementation of healthcare policy should begin with the reference to basic figures presenting the number of infections, deaths and vaccinations. The data included in this article refer to the state as of 20 June 2021 according to the John Hopkins University database (Table 4.1).

Chart 4.1 clearly shows that while the first wave of the pandemic was very mild, in the second wave particularly high increases in the number of deaths were recorded in the Czech Republic and Hungary, and the third wave brought Hungary to the top of the list mentioned above (Our World in Data. Available from: https://ourworldindata.org/covid-deaths).

The analysis of the so-called Containment and Health Index (COVID-19: Stringency Index, Our World in Data, https://ourworldindata.org/covid-stringency-index) also does not give clear answers as to why such a development occurred. This index takes into account the response to coronavirus in various areas and types of action, such as closures of schools, workplaces, travel bans, testing policies, contact tracing, face covering and vaccination rates (Chart 4.2).

As can be seen from the above data, Hungary, for example, reacted strongly during the third wave of the pandemic, introducing strict restrictions, but the results achieved were not entirely effective or satisfactory. There is much to suggest that one of the reasons for the high number of deaths may have been insufficient COVID testing and shallow or no so-called epidemic investigation. Hungary, despite the high number of deaths, was for a long time very far behind in the ranking of tests performed per population during the third wave of the pandemic (Vaski, 2021). One of the arguments raised is also the poorer health of the Hungarian population, which translates into life expectancy.

While Poland ranks better than the Czech Republic and Hungary in relation to most of the data indicated above, a completely new light on the assessment of how a country coped with the pandemic is given by the statistic showing the number of all deaths during the pandemic compared to

*Table 4.1* Selected data on the course of the pandemic in the V4 countries

| No. | Country | No. of cases | No. of deaths | No. of second-dose vaccinations | Second-dose vaccinations (%) |
|-----|---------|--------------|---------------|----------------------------------|------------------------------|
| 1 | Czech Republic | 1,665,961 | 30,278 | 2,479,001 | 23.23 |
| 2 | Poland | 2,878,634 | 74,823 | 10,993,055 | 28.95 |
| 3 | Slovakia | 391,248 | 12,478 | 1,238,271 | 22.70 |
| 4 | Hungary | 807,428 | 29,950 | 4,360,313 | 44.63 |

Source: Authors' own elaboration based on Johns Hopkins University CSSE COVID-19 Data, Our World in Data. Available from: https://ourworldindata.org/covid-deaths, accessed: June 2021.

7-day rolling average. For some countries the number of confirmed deaths is much lower than the true number of deaths. This is because of limited testing and challenges in the attribution of the cause of death.

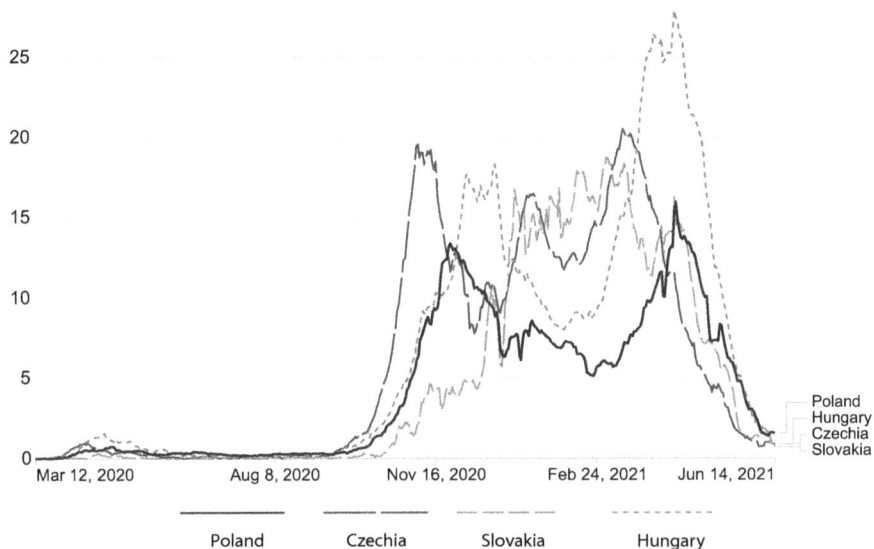

*Chart 4.1* Daily new confirmed COVID-19 deaths per million people.

Source: Johns Hopkins University CSSE COVID-19 Data, Our World in Data. Available from: https://ourworldindata.org/covid-deaths, accessed: June 2021, CC BY.

This is a composite measure based on thirteen policy response indicators including school closures, workplace closures, travel bans, testing policy, contact tracing, face coverings, and vaccine policy rescaled to a value from 0 to 100 (100 = strictest). If policies vary at the subnational level, the index is shown as the response level of the strictest sub-region.

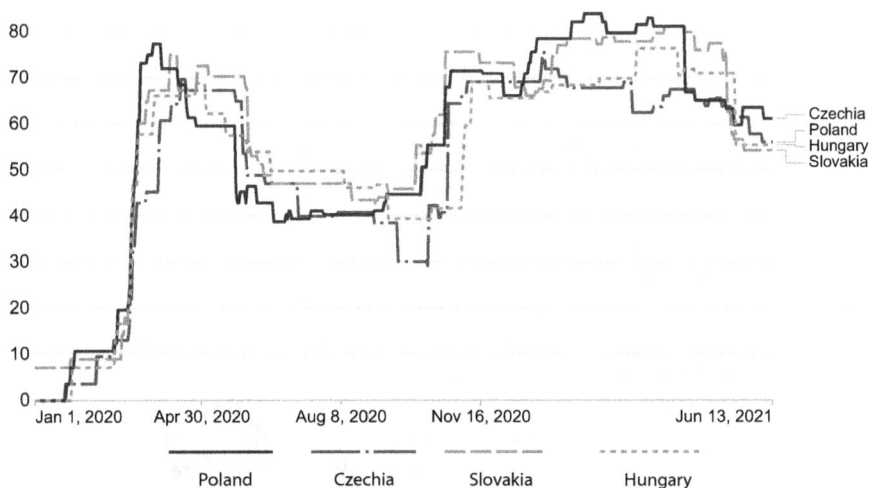

*Chart 4.2* COVID-19: Containment and Health Index.

Source: Johns Hopkins University CSSE COVID-19 Data, Our World in Data. Available from: https://ourworldindata.org/covid-deaths, accessed: June 2021, CC BY.

The percentage difference between the reported number of weekly or monthly deaths in 2020–2022 and the average number of deaths in the same period over the years 2015–2019. The reported number might not count all deaths that occurred due to incomplete coverage and delays in reporting.

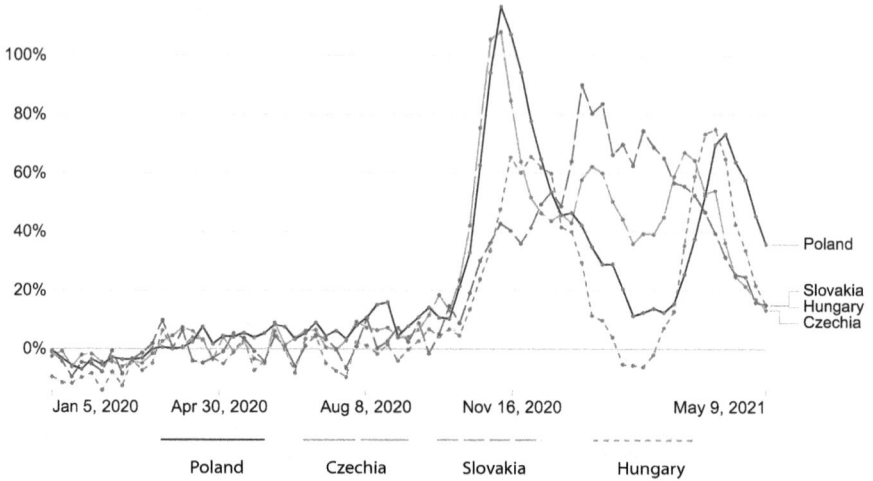

*Chart 4.3* Excess mortality: Deaths from all causes compared to previous years.

Source: Johns Hopkins University CSSE COVID-19 Data, Our World in Data. Available from: https://ourworldindata.org/covid-deaths, accessed: June 2021, CC BY.

the years 2015–2019. Analysing this data, it turns out that during both the second and third waves of the pandemic, it was Poland that recorded the highest number of "excess" deaths (Excess mortality – statistics 2021). Slovakia, which at first sight was less affected than Hungary and the Czech Republic, also recorded a very high number of deaths that exceeded the norm between the second and first waves, being then the clear, infamous V4 leader in this respect (Chart 4.3).

Pandemic forecasts for the V4 countries on the basis of assumed event scenarios, developed by the Institute for Health Metrics and Evaluation (IHME), offer an opportunity to overcome problems in healthcare policy and increase public health spending (IHME, 2021). However, it should be strongly emphasised that the scale of problems in the health sector faced by the V4 countries has exceeded the capacity of these systems. This is due to several fundamental issues.

First, healthcare expenditures in the V4 countries were (and still are) significantly lower than in the developed world. Between Poland and Hungary, and many countries of the so-called old Union, the difference is close to double. The closest to the level of these countries is the Czech Republic, which spends slightly more on healthcare than Spain and 1.4% of GDP more than Ireland. In 2019, healthcare expenditures calculated as a share of GDP were 4.3% in Poland, 4.4% in Hungary, 5.6% in Slovakia and 6.5% in the Czech Republic, while at the same time the UK spent 8%, falling slightly behind countries such as the Netherlands, Denmark, Sweden,

France and Germany (Skóbel et al., 2021). Although health spending in the V4 countries increased between 2015 and 2019, it was not enough to significantly change their position in the European ranking.

Second, investment in public health research falls short of global standards. Research work on infectious diseases has also not been significantly funded in the V4 countries. In countries with lower levels of economic development, spending on efficiency measures and innovation is often seen as a cost for which there is no budgetary space. This is a significant mistake, because these expenses are of an investment nature, which is the strength of the economy. The opportunity for the V4 countries lies in the European funds that will be allocated to increase the efficiency of healthcare systems. Another area of potential cost-effectiveness should be the restructuring of internal (national) budget expenditure on public health.

Third, the V4 countries are experiencing a shortage of specialised medical staff needed to effectively fight the pandemic. Slovak expert Miriama Letanovec Svetkovská stresses that the pandemic crisis has revealed shortages when it comes to medical staff resources. She adds that "nobody was prepared for a pandemic, but the problem of staff shortages was well known since 2010. This is what happens when no reforms are made during a period of growth" (Gabrizova, 2021). Similar accusations can also be made towards government decision-makers in the other V4 countries. In Poland, the problems of medical staff have been known *de facto* since the beginning of the political transformation, and have been exacerbated by the increased emigration of doctors and nurses in the first decade of the 21st century. The lack of an adequate number of specialised medical staff made it necessary to rapidly replenish the workforce by engaging additional staff including self-employed nurses, retired employees, final year medical students and other health-related majors such as nursing or paramedics (Pandemic Covid-19, 2020, p. 10). The Czech authorities have decided to ban the use of leave by medical staff needed to fight the pandemic (Pandemic Covid-19, 2020, p. 10). As the pandemic developed and the vaccination campaign was launched, it was decided to include more groups representing medical professions, for example, pharmacists and feldshers, in the vaccination of citizens.

Fourth, the V4 countries do not have adequate expert and technological resources for a rapid response in terms of health policy. In the V4 countries, most medical companies have been privatised, depriving them of access to fast-track research. Experts point out that in terms of innovation, the V4 countries still have a considerable distance to the most developed countries in the world and the EU (Gołębiowska, 2020a). A standardised measure used to assess the level of innovative activity of a given country is GERD (gross domestic expenditure on research and development). It measures the total national expenditure on R&D performed in the territory of a given country, incurred by the following sectors: business, government, higher education and private non-commercial institutions. Outlays of the V4 countries in terms of GERD measure are presented in Table 4.2.

Table 4.2 Gross domestic expenditure on R&D (GERD) in billion EUR in V4 countries and on average in EU28

| | 2008 | 2009 | 2010 | 2011 | 2012 | 2013 | 2014 | 2015 | 2016 | 2017 | 2018 | 2018/2008 in % |
|---|---|---|---|---|---|---|---|---|---|---|---|---|
| Poland | 2.19 | 2.10 | 2.61 | 2.84 | 3.43 | 3.44 | 3.86 | 4.32 | 4.11 | 4.83 | 6.02 | 175.00 |
| Czech Republic | 2.00 | 1.92 | 2.10 | 2.55 | 2.88 | 3.00 | 3.09 | 3.25 | 2.96 | 3.43 | 4.01 | 100.00 |
| Hungary | 1.06 | 1.07 | 1.13 | 1.20 | 1.26 | 1.42 | 1.43 | 1.51 | 1.37 | 1.67 | 2.05 | 93.00 |
| Slovakia | 0.30 | 0.30 | 0.42 | 0.47 | 0.59 | 0.61 | 0.67 | 0.94 | 0.63 | 0.75 | 0.75 | 150.00 |
| UE28 average | 8.57 | 8.48 | 8.82 | 9.28 | 9.64 | 9.79 | 10.19 | 10.79 | 10.89 | 11.43 | 12.02 | 40.00 |

Source: Authors' own elaboration based on Gołębiowska, M., Jak rozpędzić gospodarkę, czyli polityki innowacyjne państw Grupy Wyszehradzkiej. Prace IES, Lublin, 2020, p. 38.

The above data clearly indicate that although the V4 countries are taking measures to increase innovation, the gap between them and the EU average is still significant.

Fifth, in the V4 countries, a significant problem is the low level of citizens' trust in the state and its institutions and the non-compliance with the recommendations of public authorities. For example, in Slovakia, the Roma minority in the Spiš region was placed under compulsory quarantine in April 2020. This was the result of insubordination on the part of this minority which, despite knowing they were infected, moved around the country, increasing the transmission of the virus. In order to limit the mobility of the Roma, it was decided to use the Slovak army, which led to a temporary political crisis. However, this helped to limit the transmission of the virus (Koźbiał, 2021). Also in Poland and the Czech Republic various actions and protests were organised to express dissatisfaction with the introduction of restrictions and limitations.

Sixth, the Polish experience (which also affected other V4 countries) in collecting and presenting pandemic data also revealed shortcomings related to information systems supporting crisis and epidemic management. The lack of reference database systems combined with low-quality IT equipment and the lack of digital competence of sanitary inspection staff was exposed by a high school student from Toruń, who aggregated data from field units on a daily basis and presented it on a portal he had created. This data was used in the first period of the pandemic by most stakeholders in the field.

Seventh, the problem with the broader health policy of the V4 countries is the lack of a strategic management culture. In fact, it could be argued that there has been a management collapse in the public health sector. This problem should also be compounded by the lack of effective mechanisms to address conflicts of interest. Most often, the position of minister of health is held by a representative of the medical community. Thus, his perspective on the perception and evaluation of problems and their diagnosis is fraught with a high risk of management errors. Many ministers of health, representing a particular area of medicine, focused their activities on that particular area, omitting other, from their perspective less attractive ones. This leads to the bold conclusion that the minister of health should be a public health manager, not a physician. Combining managerial competence with appropriate financial, human and organisational resources may bring positive effects. In Poland, during the pandemic, the function of the minister of health was entrusted to a doctor of economics and a specialist in public management. The assessment of his performance is largely positive, which should be seen as a good omen for the period after the pandemic.

In order to fight pandemics efficiently, it is necessary to ensure a relatively permanent and sustainable stock of diverse reserves in the health system. Experts draw attention to the need to provide not only medical equipment (respirators, medical masks, etc.) and diagnostic equipment (specialised laboratories, transport equipment, tests), personal protective equipment for medical personnel, but also human resources, information systems and beds (Golinowska & Zabdyr-Jamróz, 2020). It is also necessary to carry out educational activities among the public and conduct exercises involving both the public authorities and the scientific sector, as well as business and non-governmental organisations.

The pandemic has shown how important it is also for the civil services responsible for combating the pandemic to cooperate with uniformed services. In practically all countries of the world, they played an important role in the fight against the pandemic. They participated in the construction of field hospitals and other facilities necessary to fight the pandemic, supported civilian medical staff in the implementation of patient transport, supported local authorities in providing food for the elderly and excluded, controlled compliance with quarantine and participated in the process of vaccinating the population. The potential of the Territorial Defence Forces was also used in Poland. It is also important to highlight the involvement of NGOs, which assisted the governments at various stages of the pandemic. They participated in many processes to support medics on the front line of the fight against coronavirus.

The functioning of the V4 countries during the pandemic allows us to conclude that the logistical processes supporting the fight against the pandemic were carried out efficiently. The system of organisation of vaccinations in Poland (despite some temporary problems) should be assessed positively. Such an opinion was also formulated by the president of the European Commission, Ursula von der Leyen, who indicated that Poland has been effectively implementing this process. It is also worth noting that despite their own problems and challenges, the V4 countries carried out actions aimed at supporting other countries affected by the pandemic (Czarnecki, 2020).

The pandemic, within the health policy dimension, also revealed significant problems related to the necessary medical resources. The V4 countries were fully dependent on external supplies during the initial period of the pandemic, which significantly affected the ability to ensure the safety of key medical personnel and limit virus transmission. It also revealed the lack of preparedness of many public health entities to deal with the coronavirus crisis. Medical and administrative staff were not prepared to function in such a difficult situation. This conclusion applies to all V4 countries. The above observations can be fully applied to healthcare systems that were largely focused on achieving and increasing cost efficiency. A lack of financial resources for provisioning combined with a lack of structural investment led to large deficits that could not be addressed within a few months. Years of neglect require many years of work by all stakeholders in the health system. Importantly, this must take place within the framework of a cross-party agreement, as healthcare policy cannot be the subject of a partisan political struggle and requires a long-term strategy that transcends the horizon of one political party or another in power.

One of the strategies of the V4 countries for the coming months, and perhaps even years, should be a vaccination policy based on a steady increase in vaccination rates. After the initial euphoria and anticipation of vaccines, we are currently witnessing a dangerous trend of avoiding vaccination. This is particularly risky in the context of the next wave of the pandemic, which is likely to arrive in the autumn of 2021. WHO experts are speaking in a similar tone. The highest vaccination rates among citizens are recorded in Hungary, which owes much to the use of controversial vaccines from the East, from Russia and China, among others. Although these vaccines are not authorised by the EMA for use in the EU, this has not affected the Hungarian authorities' decisions. The issues of purchasing vaccines not approved in the EU were also the cause of political crisis in Slovakia and the Czech Republic (Czarnecki et al., 2021). Prime Minister Igor Matovič decided to purchase Sputnik V vaccines, which led to clear social divisions (Lewkowicz, 2021). The other V4 countries oscillate around 30% vaccinated with the full dose. The V4 countries need to intensify their efforts to increase interest in vaccination and to clearly and immediately stigmatise fake news and disinformation activities, especially those carried out by individuals and organisations with authority among different social groups. Disinformation is also faced by other V4 countries, which confirms how important this problem is (Mesežnikov & Bartoš, 2020).

Summarising, it should be stated that the V4 countries were not well prepared for the threat posed by an infectious disease. The legal solutions in place were not adequate for the emerging challenges resulting from the dynamic spread of the virus. The legislative authorities took a number of legislative steps, but these were not always effective, consistent with the intention, or implemented at the right time. A number of pieces of legislation can be cited that have failed to achieve their purpose and have exacerbated confusion among key stakeholders. In the health policy dimension, similar conclusions can be drawn. The long-standing policy aimed at increasing the cost-effectiveness of V4 countries' healthcare systems has revealed the scale of neglect. It relates both to the issue of providing modern medical equipment, availability of professional medical staff and expenditure on research and development of medicine and even to equipping infectious disease hospitals with adequate personal protective equipment for the personnel. The lack of a clear and explicit strategy of this structure both at the V4 level and at the EU level was also significant for the assessment of the effectiveness and efficiency of the activities of the V4 countries.

However, it is important to note that the coronavirus pandemic contributed to an increase in the pace of digitisation of the V4 countries and allowed the development of effective mechanisms of cooperation among state institutions and representatives of the private sector and NGOs. In each of the V4 countries, the potential of enterprises was used to fight the pandemic and its consequences. The hypothesis assumed in the introduction of this chapter has been confirmed. Undoubtedly, the coronavirus pandemic presented the V4 countries with the greatest challenges in their modern history. Undeniably, the pandemic has affected the processes and mechanisms of functioning of the state, public decision-making and public management, moving them from a largely analogue world to a "digital world". At this stage, it is difficult to say unequivocally how the V4 countries passed this test. Some of the effects of the coronavirus pandemic will only become apparent in a few years or so. The fight against the pandemic has caused the V4 countries to incur a so-called health debt. The number of medical services provided has fallen, diagnostics have been discontinued for long periods and scheduled treatments have been cancelled en masse. It can be concluded that the efforts of the health system were diverted to the fight against the pandemic. However, it should not be forgotten that this "debt" will have to be repaid by increasing expenditure on healthcare policy. In addition, it is difficult today to estimate the scale of demand for health services that will be generated by the "recovered" people dealing with the long-term complications of the disease. We do not have much time, as the effects may be irreversible and the timing of repayment of the "debt" quicker than expected.

An unintended but very important consequence of the pandemic is the increased public confidence in the wider public health sector workers. Examples of heroic actions by medical personnel are provided by each of the countries analysed. One should hope that this trend will become permanent in these countries and not just a passing "fashion". The authors' hope is also that the authority of science and research will increase. Without proper collaboration between theoreticians and practitioners (politicians and medical personnel), major health policy challenges cannot be solved. Cooperation across divides is essential to prevent future pandemics. There is a lot of truth in the statement that the preparation phase of a pandemic is always cheaper than the response phase, and this applies to any type of threat. In political terms, a major problem is the inadequate perception and assessment of health security risks by policy makers. Surprisingly, decisions to increase defence spending are taken more quickly than health spending.

According to experts, from the beginning of the pandemic in Poland (however, this conclusion can be extrapolated to other V4 countries),

> the difficulties of the authorities in rationalising the process of planning and implementing interventions were evident. The problem was to construct a clear, coherent and logical model of intervention, to articulate the assumptions on which the sequence of activities was based, to 'translate' the intervention into a system of measurable indicators which would describe well the change the intervention aims to achieve.
>
> (Nowak & Zybała, 2020, p. 21)

There is no doubt that the V4 countries need to carry out in-depth reforms of their healthcare systems. However, it is important to remember that the reform of this sector should be a process of continuous system improvement. It should be planned, monitored and modified to adapt to the changing reality. The pandemic has highlighted a number of weaknesses and challenges, but these do not fully exhaust the problems in this area. These need to be properly diagnosed and plan mechanisms for solving them. Without this, it will not be possible to improve the quality of public health services.

## 4.3 Computerisation of the state, public services and key decision-making processes

It should be noted at the outset that the analysis covers the processes of computerisation of the state and public administration. Issues related to the computerisation of the V4 economies remain outside of consideration. In this respect, empirical data differ from data on the computerisation of the state and public administration, which will be discussed later.

The introduction of successive restrictions on social mobility has forced the states to make a kind of migration to cyberspace. UN experts rightly emphasise that e-government during the pandemic has increased its role as an indispensable element of communication, leadership and cooperation between policy makers and the public. Modern digital technologies have allowed for greater sharing of knowledge than ever before, encouraging collaboration on research related to the search for a vaccine against COVID-19, as well as improving international crisis management. For it must be remembered that viruses know no borders. This makes close international cooperation essential (MacKenzie, 2020). The same technologies designed to ensure the continuity of states and their key processes and economies have also been used to spread fake news and commit crimes in the digital space. There were hundreds of thousands of examples of hostile actions by hackers during the pandemic period. Economic crime has largely shifted to the digital world. Since the outbreak of the pandemic, cybercriminals, using a variety of tools and techniques, have robbed thousands if not millions of people. The trend of increasing cybercrime has accelerated sharply in the last several months. The same phenomena have occurred in other V4 countries. Despite the identified risks, one has to agree with the UN experts who believe that "the benefits of using technology seem to outweigh its drawbacks".[5]

There is also no doubt that the pandemic forced changes in the processes of state governance in virtually all dimensions. These changes involved both the central and local levels. Every crisis requires appropriate action. The state cannot cease to function because of restrictions on movement or on holding meetings of the legislative and executive bodies of the state. The first challenge faced by the V4 countries during the pandemic was to ensure the continuity of governance and law-making processes and public decision-making. One can venture to say that none of the V4 countries were prepared for the need to immediately migrate processes to digital space.

As part of monitoring the level of digital sophistication of the EU Member States, the European Commission has been publishing the Digital Economy and Society Index (DESI) since 2014. The latest 2020 report shows that all EU countries have seen an increase in digitisation rates over the past year. The EU digitisation leaders are Finland, Sweden and Denmark. The V4 countries occupy distant positions. The highest position – although below the EU average – is occupied by the Czech Republic (17th position). Poland is in fourth last position, ahead of Greece, Romania and Bulgaria. Details are presented in a graphic form in Chart 4.4.

The COVID-19 pandemic has also resulted in an increase in digital adoption rates across Europe. The digital adoption rate rose from 81% to 95% over the past year. According to the McKinsey study, the state of epidemic emergency has also reduced the significant differences that existed among European countries in terms of online activity. The EGDI (E-Government Development Index) published by the United Nations also increased once again in 2020. In 2018, it was 0.7926, while now it is already 0.8531. In the ranking of digital administrations, Poland is ranked 24th in the world. The other V4 countries occupy more distant positions: the Czech Republic – 39, Slovakia – 48 and Hungary – 52 (Government Survey, 2020, p. 51).

Based on the available data, one can state that

> generally, the pandemic has forced a greater demand for digital reliance across the board, and this outcome is likely here to stay in the "new normal" as the utility of more abundant data and the lowering transaction costs of using that data impact how entrepreneurs, policy-makers and professionals make decisions.
>
> (Digital trends in Europe…, 2021)

During the pandemic period, the number of domains registered with key words related to the epidemic situation such as "COVID" or "coronavirus" increased significantly. One of the reasons for this was certainly the exponentially increasing number of people seeking information about the pandemic, COVID-19 disease symptoms and treatment options. At the same time, an analysis of the available information sources showed that many websites were set up for purely disinformation activities or to carry out criminal activities.

Not only public services have been migrated to the digital space. Decision-making processes, including parliamentary, state and local government decision-making, have also been computerised. This has not been without problems resulting from the lack of adequate infrastructure, financial resources and human resources, but certainly the decision-making processes of the V4 countries have allowed the continuity of the state and its institutions. This factor should be evaluated positively, as the inability to implement decision-making processes could paralyse state activities in many areas. As has been shown many times in this study, none of the countries was (and is) prepared for such an extensive and long-lasting pandemic. The process of familiarisation with modern technologies was forced, but its effects are positive. It should be noted that the implemented solutions were

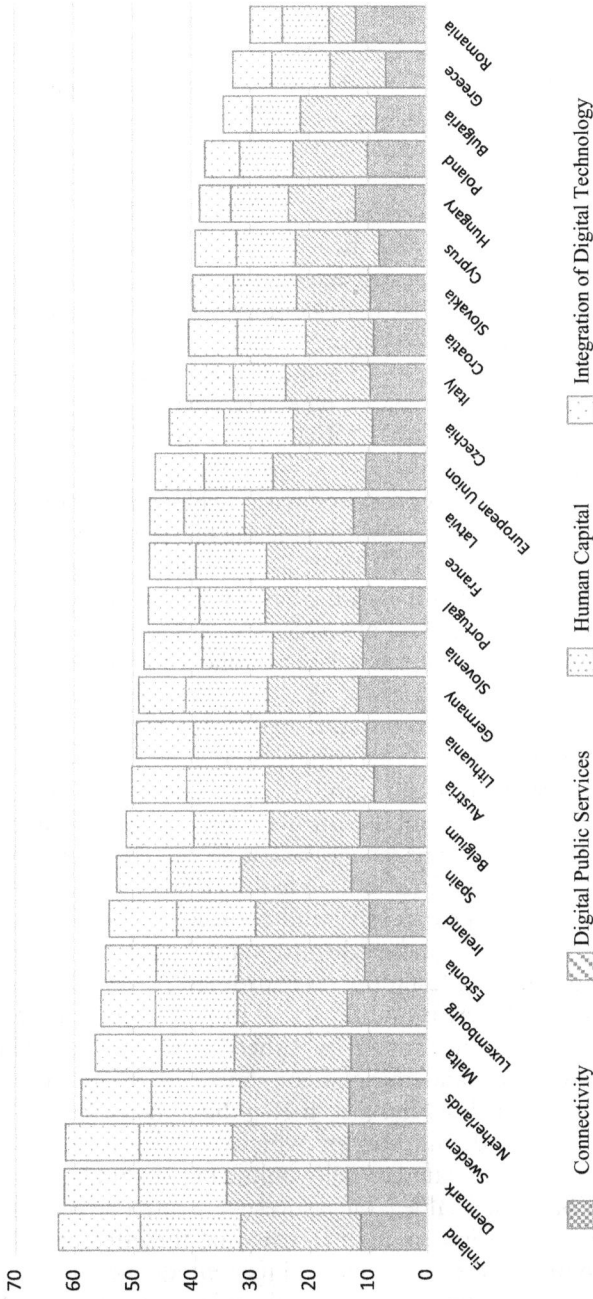

*Chart 4.4* The Digital Economy and Society Index (DESI) 2020.

Source: The Digital Economy and Society Index (DESI) 2020, European Commission. Available from: https://ec.europa.eu/digital-single-market/en/desi, accessed: 30.06.2021, CC BY

not always properly audited in terms of safety. There have been situations where unauthorised people have connected to meetings of public authorities or their proceedings have been disrupted by hackers.

Activities related to digitisation of the broadly understood health sector were extremely important. Very efficiently and quickly tools were developed to support the detection of persons in contact with patients with COVID-19, the possibility of fulfilling e-prescriptions, or schedule a remote appointment, and in the next stage, vaccination appointments. The latter has resulted in an efficient and de-bureaucratised vaccination process, for example, in Poland (Poles in Germany ..., 2021). The V4 countries have also taken steps to design and implement integrated databases for efficient and effective information and knowledge management. A number of applications were developed to improve daily contact between citizens and other stakeholders in the public health system.[6]

The pandemic also affected the education system at every level of the school system. Within days, students were forced to educate themselves using remote communication tools. Globally, more than 1.2 billion students were out of school at the peak of the pandemic (The COVID-19 pandemic..., 2020) This situation was undoubtedly a challenge for both schools and parents. There is no doubt that the pandemic has changed the country's education systems forever (The COVID-19 pandemic ..., 2020).The benefit of the pandemic may be the enforced increase in digital competence, both among students and teachers. Remote education and the use of tools supporting education in the digital space has become a permanent feature of the functioning of the V4 countries.

The accelerated digitisation of the state and its institutions has led to an intensification of activities by cybercriminals and other interest groups, including countries such as Russia and China, among others, aimed at spreading false information about the coronavirus, activities undertaken by other states and their institutions, and aimed at negatively impacting financial markets and the political situation. Virtually all countries, including the V4, have been forced to take extensive and coordinated action to counter the spread of fake news and conduct disinformation activities.

In Poland, one of the manifestations of coordinated preventive and educational activities was the creation of a social project #FakeHunter, which assumes the role of verifying content published online and exposing false information related to the pandemic and counteracting its negative effects.[7] In other V4 countries, such as the Czech Republic, the project E-Bezpečí (E-Safety) was established, the aim of which is prevention, education, research and taking action related to risky online behaviour. In Hungary, as was already mentioned, special legal measures were introduced to sanction the dissemination of false information threatening the effectiveness of the government's response to the pandemic and its consequences.

A full analysis of the actions taken and projects implemented goes beyond the intentions of the authors. However, it is necessary to draw attention to the benefits of developing public e-services. The use of public e-services on a large scale also eliminates the need for stakeholders to provide data that a public institution possesses or can obtain itself from sources it has access to. Such an activity is beneficial both for public offices and the stakeholders of the public administration system, increasing the positive perception of the level of stakeholder service.

The Visegrad countries have, to a large extent, seized the opportunity for accelerated digitisation of state structures and public services, which is evidenced by the already mentioned rankings and research results. Paradoxically, the negative impact of the pandemic on the health sector and the economy may be a turning point in the digital transformation of the Visegrad Group countries and, more broadly, Central Europe. The coronavirus pandemic has forced the V4 countries to accelerate the development of digital services. One can venture to say that this opportunity has been seized, as evidenced by the UN international rankings.

According to the authors of this chapter, there is no return to the "paper" or "analogue" state. The coronavirus pandemic has changed the public's attitude towards the computerisation of public services and e-government. "COVID impulse" has also changed the attitude of subsequent segments of the administration and institutions of the state. Computerisation has become a necessity to maintain the continuity of the state and public authority. More services provided to stakeholders had to be – due to pandemic constraints – computerised and moved to the digital space. Service recipients realised that digital service delivery could be secure, fast and time-efficient. The positive effects of the coronavirus pandemic on the computerisation of the state and public administration will stay with us permanently. IT security experts draw attention to the issue of operational digital resilience of the state. This is the ability to provide "resilience to all types of information and communication technology (ICT) related threat disruptions" (ECO/536, 2020). Undoubtedly, the pandemic has contributed to the digital resilience of the V4 countries. The scale of the challenges and problems has necessitated the development of cooperation mechanisms both within the public authority system and the public sector with representatives of business and NGOs.

The current trend should be maintained at all costs, as it may have a positive impact on the structure of spending on the public sector in the V4 countries. Undoubtedly, the mass delivery of services using remote communication tools will contribute to the reduction of employment in the wider public administration. The post-pandemic public administration and, more broadly, the post-pandemic state, must change the paradigm of functioning. In the authors' opinion, this paradigm can be called "digital centralisation of services". Its premise is as follows: the recipients of public services are in fact not interested in which body (government or local government), with which territorial jurisdiction, will deliver their service. For the recipient of a public service (just as for a bank customer) it is not important which office will realise their request. What matters is that the request is fulfilled quickly, professionally and cost-effectively.

The benefits and admiration of the efficiency of the state and its institutions in the public space must not dull our vigilance in the context of investments in the development of cyber security. Recent actions by cybercriminals, often acting on behalf of the Russian Federation or Chinese authorities, should reinforce the joint efforts of the V4 countries and the wider EU to cooperate on cyber security. Hacking attacks can be used both to take control of the state's key processes and critical infrastructure and to influence democratic processes, as was the case in the 2016 US elections (Background to "Assessing Russian...", 2017). They can also be used for disinformation activities and "steering" topics politically. It is essential to learn the lessons of the COVID-19 pandemic in the cybersecurity dimension. The pandemic can be a giant case study for designing effective mechanisms to fight crime in the digital space (Slade, 2021).

Accelerated computerisation of the state, public services and decision-making processes, as well as the economy and education, may be a significant opportunity in the development of the V4 countries. However, one should remember that the computerisation of the state and its services will have broader – systemic – consequences. This is largely due to a paradigm shift in the functioning of public administration and, more broadly, the state. During the pandemic, many public e-services were designed and implemented. As a rule, they were created at the level of central authorities. The participation of local administration was much lower, which is a result of both its legislative competences and limited financial, organisational and human resources. The emergence of many centrally managed public e-services results in natural stripping of competences of the units of the public administration system. There is no justification for maintaining duplicated resources in different institutions. Such a model of functioning of the post-pandemic e-state and e-government allows one to ask whether the dominant paradigm in the coming years will be digital centralisation of the state, while limiting the authority of local (territorial) units.

From the perspective of the efficiency and effectiveness of the functioning of the state – as evidenced by numerous examples from business – such a model is fully rational. Services are managed according to a well-known standard with maximum efficiency and effectiveness in terms of cost and time. Such an approach will be beneficial for citizens and the economy because – from their perspective – it is crucial that services provided are professional, cheap and fast. The lack of need to appear in person in an office, and thus the temporal optimisation of state stakeholders, will also be a benefit. However, the development of the e-state will have consequences related to the need to change the current model of the bureaucratic state, with its baggage of experiences and interests. It is obvious that public decision-makers who may be affected by the changes will be unhappy with this fact and will take measures to limit the process. It seems, however, that such attitudes will not gain social acceptance or will even be eliminated from public life. This is because citizens have quickly become accustomed to the fact that many public services can be provided using a mobile phone with Internet access.

The computerisation of the state and its services raises other questions. These include the use of public trust institutions, such as banks or insurers, in the provision of public services. In Poland, the use of banking sector institutions in building a modern state and public services is noticeable and important. With the use of the infrastructure of banks we can realise many public services such as establishing a trusted profile and submitting applications to various public institutions. The role of these entities – according to the authors – will continue to grow, which may also generate risks, for example, of transferring sensitive data abroad.

Regardless of the problems identified in the times of the pandemic related to the implementation of modern e-services in the V4 countries and transferring decision-making processes to digital space, it should be stated that efficient activities in this area allowed for maintaining continuity of the state's operations.

According to Łukasz Marganski of Boston Consulting Group Platinion in Central and Eastern Europe, "so far, we have only experimented with digitisation. However, we have still remained at the bottom of the pile of European countries in terms of the level of digitisation" (Oljasz, 2020).

The literature rightly notes that "social distance constraints have forced the world, among other things, to accelerate 'lessons' in connectivity, digital skills, online activities, enterprise computerisation and digital public services". Marlena Gołębiowska believes that the pandemic may paradoxically be a turning point in the digitisation process of Central European countries in the coming years (Gołębiowska, 2020b).

The literature highlights the emergence of a new regulatory paradigm as a result of the pandemic, defined as the "gold standard" for cooperation between regulators and policy makers. This paradigm aims to accelerate digital transformation horizontally. This new paradigm, according to experts from the International Telecommunication Union, "is embodied in collaborative regulation, which must engage a broad and diverse range of stakeholders in informed, evidence-based rulemaking and decision making, with both social and economic impact in mind – and with priority granted to the latter" (Digital trends in Europe, 2021). The "gold standard" paradigm can bring many benefits but often current political and economic objectives have inhibited action in this regard. One can hope that the pandemic will highlight the undeniable benefits of cooperation in the further development of digital states and societies.

Clearly, one can agree with a statement that digital transformation is a game changer – especially in "the new normal" amid the current global pandemic (Digital trends in Europe, 2021). The V4 countries can use the pandemic as a game changer in terms of the computerisation of the state and its institutions, public services and decision-making processes. The effectiveness of these activities may be enhanced if the synergy effects from cooperation within the Visegrad Group formula can be exploited. Building a modern state using the latest technologies and IT solutions will also contribute to the economic growth and, as will be discussed in the next subsection of the chapter, to increased efficiency of information and data management in the public health sector.

## 4.4 Determinants (vectors) of state-business cooperation in combating the pandemic and its consequences

The response of the V4 countries to the COVID-19 pandemic crisis in the sphere of macroeconomic action was extremely rapid and decisive. It can be said that during the pandemic crisis, the right lessons were learned from the actions and inactions following the 2007–2009 economic collapse, where many actions taken were "too little, too late". The coronavirus pandemic undoubtedly changed the paradigm of the state's cooperation with the banking sector and the business environment. One may venture to say that states and business (and especially the financial sector) have clearly tightened the iron grip that unites them, stemming from the need to develop and, in many areas, strengthen their cooperation in view of the uncertainties arising from global pandemic developments. In the initial period of the pandemic, business representatives, and in particular the banking sector, expected the state and its institutions to take measures to increase the stability of the banking sector, on the one hand, and to take action to allow key sectors of the affected economies to function, on the other. This trend was observed in virtually all countries in the world.

In the context of the issue at hand, it can also be mentioned that practically in all countries affected by the pandemic an increased role of public enterprises (SOEs) can be observed, which has been pointed out, among others, by OECD experts. These enterprises have been in many cases mobilised by the state owner (shareholder) for activities such as production and transport of sanitary materials, people or provision of infrastructure for field hospitals – with these activities usually being compensated from the state budget. Moreover, the pandemic has increased interest in increasing state participation or renationalisation in key sectors. For example, in Poland the largest companies with Treasury shareholding carried out significant activities related to, inter alia, construction of temporary hospitals (Orlen, Lotos, KGHM or PKO BP) and their maintenance, production of masks and other medical products necessary to limit transmission of the virus and production of hygienic liquids (Orlen, Lotos, ARP).

However, it is worth noting that fully private companies have also become involved in the fight against the pandemic. In the case of entities from the V4 countries, it is worth noting the involvement of companies such as the Czech Skoda, the Slovak IT company ESET, the Hungarian oil company MOL and the Polish Amica. These entities undertook various types of activities aimed at supporting the state, in particular the entities responsible for implementing healthcare policy and directly combating the pandemic. It should also be noted that the support also included the provision of cash donations and funding of scientific research to support the fight against the pandemic. However, these activities were marginal in the context of the support offered by national governments and the European Union.

On the basis of the research and analyses carried out, it may be concluded that in the V4 countries, cooperation between the state and business was limited primarily to the preparation and consultation of government aid programmes for enterprises and citizens, i.e. consumers of goods and services. This phenomenon was analogous also in relation to other countries of the world. Cooperation with business took on the dimension of, inter alia, meetings with employers' organisations or social consultations of law amendments. In this context, it can be concluded that entrepreneurs were mainly the recipients of direct assistance or benefited from changes in legislation aimed at facilitating the functioning of companies, and were also indirectly influenced by the assistance provided to citizens (potential customers). The main activities of the V4 countries aimed at entrepreneurs will be characterised below.

Restrictions introduced by governments have not always met with approval or understanding from entrepreneurs. The chapter on pandemic legislation points out that legislators have not always introduced legal solutions that responded to the needs of businesses. In particular, the industries most affected by the pandemic have flaunted their discontent. For example, restaurateurs and hotel owners have welcomed customers despite bans, manifesting their dissatisfaction with successive lockdowns. The governments' response in this regard has been protective regulations to compensate businesses for the loss of turnover and revenue associated with pandemic restrictions, while at the same time encouraging job retention.

Since 6 April 2020, the Hungarian government has been implementing the so-called Economic Defence Plan, which is based, among others, on the following pillars:

- preservation of jobs (e.g. when employing part-time workers, the government takes over part of the wage costs from employers);
- a programme to protect families and the elderly (between 2021 and 2024, pensioners will receive a 13th pension);
- relaunch of key economic sectors (tourism, construction, film and creative industries, agriculture, health, food, logistics and transport, which are supported through government-guaranteed loans – a total of around EUR 5.5 billion);
- business financing in the form of concessional loans (until 2022). A Property Protection Capital Fund has also been set up in this pillar to reduce the risk of hostile takeovers;
- creation of new jobs (in 2020, investments were supported by a total of around EUR 1.2 billion);
- tax relief and reduction of administrative burdens (including simplification of procedures, extension of deadlines and changes in tax settlements).

In addition, a total of around EUR 2.6 billion was allocated to the so-called Economic Defence Fund in 2020 and around EUR 7.3 billion for 2021. A special Operational Staff for the Defence of the Economy, chaired by the Minister of Finance, has also been established. The purpose of the staff's activities is to return Hungary to the path of rapid economic growth, to monitor the implementation of the plan for the defence of the economy and to propose the elimination of such regulations that hinder companies' activities and investments in Hungary.

Within and outside the above-mentioned programme, the government has also taken a number of measures in the form of permitted state aid (approved by the European Commission) for various sectors of the economy and the labour market. These measures are summarised synthetically in chronological order on the European Commission's website, so there is no need to cite them here (Details of Hungary's ..., 2021).

As regards the public enterprise sector, it should be mentioned that the Hungarian government is currently planning to take over Budapest Airport, motivated by strategic considerations – including the important role that airports played during the pandemic (it should be remembered that Hungary has been consistently implementing a plan to renationalise key sectors since 2010, regardless of the current situation). Moreover, as has already been mentioned, the Hungarian government has used the powers granted during the state of emergency dozens of times, concerning control over private companies (including the introduction of representatives of state power ministries) of strategic importance (which was determined on a discretionary basis) and hospitals (the military authorities took over supervision of half of them) – with the actual acquisition of a controlling stake taking place once, in the case of Kartonpack Zrt, which can be considered a political move (the plant is not medically or strategically important, and its takeover started mainly the exchange of the Board of Directors and legal disputes with shareholders).

In the Czech Republic, a government programme to support entrepreneurs, including a loan programme, has been ongoing since March 2020. In the third iteration of the programme (COVID III), still in 2020, banks have received 1,629 applications for guaranteed loans of around EUR 500 million. The funding for the programme amounts to CZK 150 billion. Self-employed persons and companies with up to 250 employees are entitled to guarantees of up to 90%, companies with up to 500 employees will receive a guarantee of up to 80%. The government expects that up to 150,000 entrepreneurs will benefit from the loans thanks to the state guarantees (COVID III..., 2020).

In addition, a programme with a budget of around EUR 7.3 million to support pandemic-related research and development activities was launched in May 2020. Funds from the programme are available to all companies in the Czech Republic that are able to carry out R&D projects in all sectors. The aim of the programme is to support the development of innovative solutions useful in combating the coronavirus, such as medical and paramedical technologies and solutions, including 3D printing systems and logistics applications.

It should also be noted that the Czech government has approved a draft amendment to the Income Tax Act in order to simplify, starting from 2021, the payment of taxes and social security contributions by small entrepreneurs and self-employed persons with annual revenues of up to CZK 800,000 (approximately EUR 32,000). These taxpayers will be able to pay one lump sum for income tax as well as social and health insurance contributions. Lump-sum taxpayers will not have to submit tax returns and insurance declarations.

In addition, within and outside the above-mentioned programme, the government has taken a number of measures in the form of permitted state aid (approved by the European Commission) for various sectors of the economy and labour market. These measures are summarised synthetically, in chronological order, on the European Commission's website (Details of Czechia's ..., 2021).

Moreover, the Czech government has cooperated with state and private companies on, among other things, the urgent construction of field hospitals, which incidentally caused controversy – e.g. in the case of the long-term lease of the Prague Expo grounds for a field hospital, which has never been used due to a shortage of medical staff.

In Slovakia, while the first waves of the pandemic were still unfolding in 2020, the government approved more than a hundred amendments to laws aimed at improving the business environment and helping to kick-start the Slovak economy after the pandemic. This activity continued into 2021. The changes included, for example: (1) simplification of permits for the construction of infrastructure (e.g. telecommunications); (2) reduced requirements for auditing reports in the case of an increase in the share capital of a limited liability company; (3) possible automatic increase in fuel consumption costs incurred, calculated according to the consumption stated in the registration certificate or technical certificate or in supplementary data from the manufacturer or dealer, by 20% without the obligation to document and specify higher fuel consumption; (4) introduction of a second chance principle (no fine) for a natural or legal person who fails to meet his/her obligation within the deadlines specified in the various provisions of the Social Security Act but then meets it within the following seven days; (5) subsidies for employers and for companies in the key sectors and tourism; and (6) guaranteed loans for, inter alia, start-ups (Details of Slovakia's..., 2021).

Within and outside the above-mentioned activities, the government has also taken a number of measures in the form of permitted state aid (approved by the European Commission) for various sectors of the economy and labour market (Details of Slovakia's..., 2021).

The Polish government has also taken a number of measures to support businesses affected by the pandemic and to protect the economy. At the beginning of April, the European Commission approved a programme which involved the Polish development bank, Bank Gospodarstwa Krajowego, providing public guarantees for investment loans and working capital for medium-sized and large Polish enterprises in all sectors. In May, a substantial programme of subsidised loans was implemented to support large enterprises in the wake of the coronavirus pandemic. This was part of a larger support programme, the so-called Financial Shield for large enterprises, which amounted to EUR 2.2 billion. A state guarantee on factoring products was also implemented, with the Commission's approval. This measure was intended to provide liquidity to the real economy as it involves the payment of invoices before their final maturity. At the end of 2020, a programme of around EUR 3 billion was adopted to support micro, small and medium-sized enterprises in certain sectors, including retail, hotels, leisure and transport, affected by the coronavirus pandemic (Details of Poland's..., 2021).

To sum up this discussion, it can be said that, despite its many negative effects, the pandemic has definitely had positive aspects. It became a kind of catalyst for constructive and reliable dialogue between the public sphere and state institutions, on the one hand, and business, on the other. This made it possible to develop many pragmatic solutions that mitigated the impact of the pandemic on economic actors. Of course, many industries have been seriously affected by the pandemic, but this problem does not only affect the V4 countries. This phenomenon is present practically all over the world.

Analysts of the Politico website, analysing the effectiveness and efficiency of the fight against the pandemic of Central European countries, pointed out that the V4 countries "share something tragic in common: They have among the worst cumulative death rates from COVID-19 in Europe, far above the EU average and above most Western European countries" (Politico..., 2021). In their view, "pandemic response was shaped by a strong preference among policymakers to opt for populist quick fixes rather than make tough calls based on science" (Politico..., 2021). This statement illustrates well the mechanisms of pandemic governance. Leaders of the V4 countries "have picked fights with public health experts for perceived political gain and cut corners when enacting pandemic regulations" (Politico..., 2021). Politicians' lack of trust in the expert and scientific communities contributed to the lower effectiveness of the undertaken measures.

## Notes

1 Cf.: e.g. Vikarská, Z., Czechs and Balances... The issue of admissibility of individual pandemic restrictions has already been the subject of judicial review in the Czech Republic, with different rulings, partly overturning, e.g. certain trade bans, and partly upholding the introduced restrictions. The question of state liability remains open, with government representatives cutting off potential compensation. The author suggests that a possible defence against damages actions may be to deny causation by showing that the damage suffered is not caused by government restrictions but by the pandemic.

2 One should bear in mind that each legal order has its own peculiarities, expressed in particular in the specific way in which extraordinary measures are framed in the constitution. For example, the Italian Constitution does not provide for an extraordinary measure, cf.: Bosek, 2021, p. 128. In this sense, the conclusions concerning the evaluation of the actions of individual governments cannot be transferred unreflectively between legal orders. Nevertheless, an attempt can be made to develop a model for evaluating the applied measures.

3 Pursuant to Article 232 of the Constitution of the Republic of Poland, the Council of Ministers may impose a state of natural disaster "in order to prevent or remove the consequences of a natural catastrophe or a technological accident exhibiting characteristics of a natural disaster". In literature it is indicated – with reference to Art. 3(1)(2) of the Act of 18 April 2002 on the state of natural disaster – that the definition of natural disaster may also include mass occurrence of infectious diseases in humans (cf.: Steinborn, 2016; Florczak-Wątor, 2020, p. 8).

4 The discussion in this respect continues not only in Poland, a current example of which is the ruling of the French Council of State of 5 August 2021, in which the Council of State held that making the use of certain services (bars, restaurants) conditional on having a sanitary certificate, as well as mandatory vaccination of medical staff, are in accordance with the French Constitution (France: Passes… 2020). As similar restrictions or obligations have been introduced in other countries (e.g. Italy), it is to be expected that other constitutional courts will also decide on analogous issues.

5 E-Government Survey 2020 Digital Government in the Decade of Action for Sustainable Development with Addendum on COVID-19 Response, United Nations, Department of Economic and Social Affairs, New York, 2020, p. 215.

6 In Poland, a dedicated website has been set up at www.gov.pl/koronawirus. This website is dedicated to the pandemic – and according to the authors' declaration – one can find reliable, verified and certain information on the epidemic situation in the country. The portal also publishes hints, tips and guidelines of sanitary services, facilitating navigation in the maze of legal regulations. The need for this action is demonstrated by the figures. In March and April 2020 the gov.pl portal was visited by almost 46 million users. Cyfryzacja podczas pandemii. Innowacje. Bezpieczeństwo. E-administracja. Wybrane działania Ministerstwa Cyfryzacji marzec – wrzesień 2020. Warszawa, 2020.

7 The project was launched by the Polish Press Agency and GovTech Poland (https://fakehunter.pap.pl).

# References

Background to "Assessing Russian … (2017). *Background to "Assessing Russian Activities and Intentions in Recent US Elections": The Analytic Process and Cyber Incident Attribution*. Office of the Director of National Intelligence, January.

Białynicki-Birula, P. (2013). Polityka ochrony zdrowia. In M. Zawicki (Ed.), *Wprowadzenie do nauk o polityce publicznej*. Warsaw: Polskie Wydawnictwo Ekonomiczne, pp. 207–225.

Biga, B. (2020). *Patolegislacja. Dlaczego pandemia nie wybaczy fuszerki?* Available from: https://klubjagiellonski.pl/2020/10/14/patolegislacja-dlaczego-pandemia-nie-wybaczy-fuszerki/

Bosek, L. (2021). Anti-Epidemic Emergency Regimes under Polish Law in Comparative. Historical and Jurisprudential Perspective. *EJHL*, 28(2), pp. 113–141. DOI: 10.1163/15718093-BJA10039

Braumberger, A. (2020). *Polacy wściekli za zakaz wstępu do lasu. Petycja nic nie dała, dalej grozi 30 tys. Kary.* Available from: https://spidersweb.pl/bizblog/zakaz-wstepu-do-lasu/

COVID III – kolejny pakiet pomocy dla czeskich firm (2020). Portal Promocji Eksportu. Available from: https://czechrepublic.trade.gov.pl/pl/aktualnosci/309424,kolejny-pakiet-pomocy-dla-czeskich-firm-.html

Current healthcare expenditure relative to GDP (2018). *Current healthcare expenditure relative to GDP.* Eurostat. Available from: https://ec.europa.eu/eurostat/statistics-explained/index.php?title=Healthcare_expenditure_statistics

Czarnecki, S. (2020). Czechy wobec COVID-19: pomoc międzynarodowa, Chiny i czeska polityka wewnętrzna. *Komentarze IEŚ*, 178(81).

Czarnecki, Sz., Hejj, D., Lewkowicz, Ł., & Tatarenko, A. (2021). Dylematy szczepionkowe państw Grupy Wyszehradzkiej. *Komentarze IEŚ*, 376(73).

Details of Czechia's Support Measures (2021). *Details of Czechia's support measures to help citizens and companies during the significant economic impact of the coronavirus pandemic.* European Commission. Available from: https://ec.europa.eu/info/live-work-travel-eu/coronavirus-response/jobs-and-economy-during-coronavirus-pandemic/state-aid-cases/czechia_en

Details of Hungary's Support Measures (2021). *Details of Hungary's support measures to help citizens and companies during the significant economic impact of the coronavirus pandemic.* European Commission. Available from: https://ec.europa.eu/info/live-work-travel-eu/coronavirus-response/jobs-and-economy-during-coronavirus-pandemic/state-aid-cases/hungary_en

Details of Poland's Support Measures (2021). *Details of Poland's support measures to help citizens and companies during the significant economic impact of the coronavirus pandemic.* European Commission. Available from: https://ec.europa.eu/info/live-work-travel-eu/coronavirus-response/jobs-and-economy-during-coronavirus-pandemic/state-aid-cases/poland_pl?etrans=pl

Details of Slovakia's Support Measures (2021*). Details of Slovakia's support measures to help citizens and companies during the significant economic impact of the coronavirus pandemic.* European Commission. Available from: https://ec.europa.eu/info/live-work-travel-eu/coronavirus-response/jobs-and-economy-during-coronavirus-pandemic/state-aid-cases/slovakia_en

Digital trends in Europe (2021). *Digital trends in Europe 2021 ICT trends and developments in Europe 2017-2020.* International Telecommunication Union.

ECO/536 (2020). Operational digital resilience, Brussels, 27 November 2020.

E-Government Survey (2020). *E-Government Survey 2020 Digital Government in the Decade of Action for Sustainable Development With addendum on COVID-19 Response.* United Nations, Department of Economic and Social Affairs, New York.

Excess Mortality – Statistics, Eurostat 2021. Available from: https://ec.europa.eu/eurostat/statistics-explained/index.php?title=Excess_mortality_-_statistics#Excess_mortality_in_the_European_Union_between_January_2020_and_April_2021

Florczak-Wątor, M. (2020). Niekonstytucyjność ograniczeń praw i wolności jednostki wprowadzonych w związku z epidemią COVID-19 jako przesłanka odpowiedzialności odszkodowawczej państwa. *Państwo i Prawo*, 75, 12(898), Warsaw, pp. 5–22.

Gabrizova, Z. (2021). *Grupa Wyszehradzka: Kto wygrał, a kto stracił na pandemii?* Available from: https://www.euractiv.pl/section/grupa-wyszehradzka/news/grupa-wyszehradzka-pandemia-koronawirus-covid-19-polska-czechy-slowacja-wegry-morawiecki-matovic-babis-orban-transformacja/

Ginsburg, T., & Versteeg, M. (2020). The Bound Executive: Emergency Powers during the Pandemic. *Virginia Public Law and Legal Theory Research Paper*, 2020-52, University of Chicago, Public Law Working Paper No. 747, available at SSRN: http://dx.doi.org/10.2139/ssrn.3608974

GHS Index (2019). *Global Health Security Index. Building Collective Action and Accountability.* Available from: https://www.ghsindex.org/wp-content/uploads/2019/10/2019-Global-Health-Security-Index.pdf

Gołębiowska, M. (2020a). *Jak rozpędzić gospodarkę, czyli polityki innowacyjne państw Grupy Wyszehradzkiej.* Lublin: Prace IEŚ.

Gołębiowska, M. (2020b). COVID-19 a cyfryzacja Europy Środkowej. *Komentarze Instytutu Europy Środkowej*, 162(65).

Golinowska, S., & Zabdyr-Jamróz, M. (2020). Zarządzanie kryzysem zdrowotnym w pierwszym półroczu pandemii COVID-19. Analiza porównawcza na podstawie opinii ekspertów z wybranych krajów. *Zdrowie Publiczne i Zarządzanie*, 18(1), pp. 1–31, DOI: 10.4467/20842627OZ.20.001.12655

Héjj, D. (2020a). Węgry w obliczu drugiej fali pandemii wirusa SARS-CoV-2. *Komentarze IEŚ*, 258(161). Available from: https://ies.lublin.pl/komentarze/wegry-w-obliczu-drugiej-fali-pandemii-wirusa-sars-cov-2/

Héjj, D. (2020b). Węgry w stanie zagrożenia. W czasie pandemii COVID-19 rząd Viktora Orbána z nadzwyczajnymi uprawnieniami. *Komentarze IEŚ*, 157(60). Available from: https://ies.lublin.pl/komentarze/wegry-w-stanie-zagrozenia-w-czasie-pandemii-covid-19-rzad-viktora-orbana-z-nadzwyczajnymi-uprawnieniami/

IHME (2021). *Prognozy COVID – IHME. Raport dla krajów Grupy Wyszehradzkiej.* IHME. Available from: https://www.aotm.gov.pl/media/2021/05/Prognozy-COVID-IHME-AOTMIT-GrupaWyszehradzka-17.05.2021.pdf

Kardas, P. (2020). Konstytucyjne podstawy rozstrzygania kolizji obowiązków i konfliktu dóbr w czasie pandemii. *Palestra*, 6(751), pp. 5–28.

Karsai, D. (2020). *The Curious and Alarming Story of the City of Göd. How the Hungarian Government misuses its power in their political fight against opposition-led municipalities.* Available from: https://verfassungsblog.de/the-curious-and-alarming-story-of-the-city-of-goed/

Koldinská, K. (2020). *COVID-19 measures – ban on presence of fathers during birth of child, Flash Report.* Available from: https://www.equalitylaw.eu/downloads/5141-czech-republic-covid-19-measures-ban-on-presence-of-fathers-during-birth-of-child-72-kb

Kośka, M. (2020). *Żądamy cofnięcia zakazu wstępu do lasu!". Ponad 125 tys. osób w dwa dni podpisało petycję.* Available from: https://www.money.pl/gospodarka/zadamy-cofniecia-zakazu-wstepu-do-lasu-ponad-125-tys-osob-w-dwa-dni-podpisalo-petycje-6496581100710017a.html

Koźbiał, K. (2021). *Analiza sytuacji na Słowacji, wystąpienie na konferencji naukowej Era COVID-19.* Ocena działań decydentów politycznych na świecie podczas pandemii, March.

Kubicka-Żach, K. (2020). *Zakaz wstępu do lasu fikcyjny? Nie ma podstaw prawnych.* Available from: https://www.prawo.pl/samorzad/przywolywane-podstawy-prawne-zakazu-wstepu-do-lasu-nie,499297.html

Kustra-Rogatka, A. (2020). *Backgrounder: Poland's presidential elections, covid-19 and the rule of law crisis.* Available from: https://democracyreporting.org/dri_publications/backgrounder-polandspresidential-elections-covid-19-and-the-rule-of-law-crisis/

Lalonde, M. (1974). *A New Perspective on the Health of Canadians; A Working Document.* Ottawa: Information Canada.

Lewkowicz, Ł. (2021). Słowacja: podejście do szczepionki Sputnik V dzieli społeczeństwo. *Komentarze IEŚ*, 381(78).

Mackenzie, D. (2020). *Covid-19: pandemia, która nie powinna była się zdarzyć i jak nie dopuścić do następnej.* Wydawnictwo Zysk i S-ka.

Mesežnikov, G., & Bartoš J. (2020). *Infodémia na Slovensku 2020. Dezinformačno-konšpiračná scéna v období COVID-19.* Available from: https://www.ivo.sk/buxus/docs/publikacie/subory/Infodemia_na_Slovensku_2020.pdf

Nowak, M.J., & Zybała, A. (2020). Polityka przestrzenna i jej uwarunkowania w okresie pandemii COVID-19. Zagrożenia, wyzwania i reakcje władz publicznych. In A. Bartoszewicz, K. Księżopolski, & A. Zybała (Eds.), *Polska… Unia Europejska… Świat… w pandemii COVID-19 – wybrane zagadnienia.* Warsaw: Dom Wydawniczy ELIPSA, pp. 19–32.

Nowicka, K. (2020). *Preparing for the pandemic elections.* Available from: https://verfassungsblog.de/preparing-for-the-pandemic-elections/

Oljasz, T. (2020). *BCG: Pandemia COVID-19 gwałtownie przyspieszy transformację cyfrową w Polsce*, Money.pl, 27.05. https://www.money.pl/gielda/bcg-pandemia-covid-19-gwaltownie-przyspieszy-transformacje-cyfrowa-w-polsce-6514973019654273a.html

Pecyna, M. (2020). Odpowiedzialność odszkodowawcza Skarbu Państwa za ograniczenia praw i wolności w czasie epidemii COVID-19. *Państwo i Prawo*, 12, pp. 23–37.

Poles in Germany Return Home for "Quicker, Less Bureaucratic" Covid Vaccines (2021). Available from: https://notesfrompoland.com/2021/05/12/poles-in-germany-return-home-for-quicker-less-bureaucratic-covid-vaccines/

Politico (2021). *Central Europe's deadly pandemic blunders*, Politico.eu. Available from: https://www.politico.eu/article/eastern-europe-visegrad-four-deadly-pandemic-blunders/

Raport COVID-owy. Z tarczą czy na tarczy? Legislacja w czasach zarazy (2020). Pracodawcy RP. Available from: https://pracodawcyrp.pl/upload/files/2020/12/raport-covid-final.pdf?utm_medium=email&utm_source=getresponse&utm_content=Legislacja+w+czasach+zarazy+–+raport+COVID-owy+Pracodawców+RP&utm_campaign=

RPO entry bans (2021). Rząd nie mógł zakazać zgromadzeń. Precedensowy wyrok SN po kasacji RPO ws. manifestacji pod biurem poselskim w związku z wyrokiem TK ws. aborcji, Rzecznik Praw Obywatelskich. Available from: https://bip.brpo.gov.pl/pl/content/rzad-nie-mogl-zakazac-zgromadzen-w-pandemii-wyrok-sn-po-kasacji-rpo

Sadurski, W. (2020). *The Polish presidential campaign in the shadow of the pandemic.* Available from: https://verfassungsblog.de/the-polish-presidential-campaign-in-the-shadow-of-the-pandemic/

Skóbel, B., Kocemba, E., & Rudka, R. (2021). *Nakłady na ochronę zdrowia w Polsce na tle innych państw OECD.* Związek Powiatów Polskich. Available from: https://zpp.pl/storage/files/2021-01//2378e507c871df3ca0f4f1e03fa61152534.pdf

Slade, R. (2021). *Cybersecurity Lessons from CoVID-19.* London: Routledge.

Śmiertelne grzechy Polski i jej sąsiadów z Europy Środkowej w walce z pandemią (2021). *Onet.pl.* Available from: https://wiadomosci.onet.pl/politico/koronawirus-umieralnosc-na-covid-w-polsce-duzo-wyzsza-niz-srednia-europejska/2l98bsb

Statistics and Research (n.d.). Coronavirus (COVID-19) Deaths, Our World in Data. Available from: https://ourworldindata.org/covid-deaths

Steinborn, S. (2016). In M. Safjan, & L. Bosek (Eds), *Konstytucja RP. Tom II. Komentarz do art. 87–243*. Legalis, Point III.1., No. 8 to Art. 232.

The COVID-19 pandemic has changed education forever. This is how, World Economic Forum (2020). Available from: https://www.weforum.org/agenda/2020/04/coronavirus-education-global-covid19-online-digital-learning/

Urbanovics, A., Sasvàri, P., & Teleki, B. (2020). *Evaluation of the COVID-19 regulations in the Visegrad group, Transforming Government: People, Process and Policy*. Available from: https://www.emerald.com/insight/1750-6166.htm

Vaski, T. (2021). *Why Did Hungary's Death Rate Increase So Drastically in the Third Wave?* Available from: https://hungarytoday.hu/hungary-third-wave-death-rate-covid-deaths-coronavirus/

Vikarská, Z. (2021). *Czechs and Balances – If the Epidemiological Situation Allows*. Available from: https://verfassungsblog.de/czechs-and-balances-if-the-epidemiological-situation-allows/

Wyrok SN I NSW 2849/20 (2020). Wyrok Sądu Najwyższego z dnia 28 lipca 2020. I NSW 2849/20, LEX No. 3043973.

Wysocki, M.J., & Miller, M. (2003). Paradygmat Lalonde`a, Światowa Organizacja Zdrowia i Nowe Zdrowie Publiczne. *Przegląd Epidemiologiczny*, 57(3), pp. 505–512. ISSN 0033-2100 E-ISSN 2545-1898

Ziółkowski, M. (2020). *An election in the time of pandemic*. Available from: https://verfassungsblog.de/an-election-in-the-time-of-pandemic/

# 5 Solving social problems during a pandemic

*Paweł Hut*

The COVID-19 pandemic triggered profound changes in the perception of social problems. Decision-makers responsible for the area of social policy have made significant re-evaluations in the implementation of previous tasks. Social problems – such as migration or climate protection, labour market protection, as well as cultural and social problems resulting from the reorganisation of social life and imposed social isolation – have become one of the biggest challenges. The focus of this chapter is the Visegrad Group countries. Their territorial scope is supported by the uniqueness of this area manifested by the common experience of the specificity of the post-totalitarian state, a similar level of economic development and economic situation, as well as a high ethnic homogeneity of the countries in the region. This chapter attempts to answer the following research questions about the Visegrad Group countries: What actions were taken during the COVID-19 pandemic? How did they change in different periods of the pandemic? How should the counteraction – in the Visegrad countries during the COVID-19 pandemic – of social problems such as migration, employment and unemployment, climate policy and solving social problems be assessed in retrospect? It is important to assess the course and similarities and differences in the activities of the authorities of individual countries.

In light of the analysis of data sources conducted so far, it can be assumed that the activities undertaken by individual governments of the Visegrad Group countries had a very diverse scope and duration of implementation. Reactivity and spontaneity, as well as individual and particularistic counteracting of the pandemic on the territory of individual states, should be considered a common element of the activities of the V4 countries.

In this chapter, the "state" is understood as a high form of organisation of society, whose aim is individually or collectively understood human welfare (Dudek et al., 2013, p. 1). This organisation of society manifests itself in the development of central and local government institutions, but also in the satisfaction of the needs of its members.

Detailed considerations will begin with a discussion of migration issues during the pandemic, followed by labour market protection and unemployment. In the following part, climate policy will be characterised, followed

DOI: 10.4324/9781003353812-6

by solutions to social problems using selected examples. In the Summary section, conclusions on the impact of the pandemic will be described.

## 5.1 Migrations during the pandemic

The announcement of the COVID-19 pandemic strongly affected migration processes. Already on 4 March 2020, at the request of the president of the Council of Ministers of the Republic of Poland, M. Morawiecki, a meeting of representatives of the Visegrad Group member states was convened in Prague, whose main topics were migration and the threat of coronavirus. During the meeting, its participants maintained their position ruling out the relocation of migrants from the southern EU States and decided to coordinate their actions in countering the epidemic.

In times of mass migration flows, countering the spread of the virus and health protection measures required drastic restrictions on the spatial mobility of citizens. Based on the decisions of authorities of individual states, the possibility of arrival of foreigners from abroad was restricted, whereas the citizens were allowed to return to their countries of origin if they remained under epidemiological surveillance for the prescribed period. Restrictions on crossing the Polish border were introduced from 27 March to 13 April 2020. At the same time, similar decisions were taken by the governments of other EU countries, including the other Visegrad Group countries.

In particular, the restrictions covered international collective air, rail and bus transport. Many services were cancelled and then suspended.[1] It was only when the number of diagnosed cases of SARS-CoV-2 infection decreased that services were resumed – however, they were no longer on the scale and in the "pre-pandemic" form but were subject to various restrictions: for example, on the number of seats allowed in a train compartment or on an aircraft.

Shortly after the declaration of the pandemic in March 2020, restrictions on cross-border movements were introduced in accordance with the individual decisions of national governments. Travellers were required to demonstrate a substantial purpose for entering the host country and to undergo quarantine after crossing the border. This phenomenon took on a particular dimension in the eastern part of the Schengen area.

In the Visegrad countries, detailed border controls were reintroduced. After 12 years, Euroregions and border towns were separated. The reapportionment of towns such as Teschen (Cieszyn) and Zhorjelc/Goerlitz (Zgorzelec) became a symbol of this period. Officers appeared at the former border crossings. Uniformed patrols prevented border crossings also on the local field and forest roads, previously blocked with concrete or sand barriers, and hiking trails in the mountains were also patrolled.

Decisions restricting entry into one's own country stemmed from a desire to halt the proliferation of the virus. Limiting international migration flows only to drivers of international cargo transport (TIR) was supposed to reduce the number of infections. It is difficult to assess whether these restrictions actually had the desired effect, but in the first period the announced "closure of borders" resulted in increased migration. Thousands of economic migrants who were temporarily employed by foreign employers suddenly decided to return to their countries of origin. The overnight suspension of air and rail connections caused a kind of panic and increased fears of being forced to stay in another country. These fears were strongest among people whose labour market status was not fully regulated, but people with permanent employment contracts also decided to leave. The collective memory is etched with traffic jams at Polish-German road border crossings, hundreds of people waiting for border checks at the Polish-Ukrainian pedestrian border crossing point at Medyka-Shegini and passengers camping at airports trying to find any connection to their country of origin.

The "Flight Home" campaign organised by the Polish government became a symbol of the chaotic activities of this period. Between 15 March and 5 April 2020, as many as 388 flights were made from 71 cities on six continents, from which approximately 25,000 Poles benefited.[2] Interested Polish citizens permanently residing abroad gained the possibility of rapid transport to Poland. At the same time, this action was met with a wave of criticism that the arrivals actually led to the spread in Polish society of a virus transmitted by more vulnerable Polish citizens residing in environments having frequent contact with Chinese citizens. Although none of the connections was direct from the People's Republic of China, people from Vietnam and other Asian countries were nevertheless taken, as well as travellers who were waiting at major airports for a connection to Poland. The flight to the country was also criticised for the high cost of the trip (about 350–500 euros/person).

Previously, similar air operations were organised by carriers from France, Germany, the Czech Republic, Latvia, Belgium, Lithuania and the UK. However, in their case, the EU civil protection mechanism was used. All willing citizens of the EU Member States were taken on board and 75% of the costs were covered by the European Commission's budget. A particular controversy was caused by the flights operated by France for people from Wuhan. As early as the last day of January 2020, around 220 people were evacuated by an Air and Space Force transport plane from Oise and quarantined on arrival. At the beginning of February 2020, a further 65 people were transported on two flights by chartered Fly Malta aircraft and another group of 38 people arrived thanks to a flight organised by the UK Government. The final group of 30 people from Wuhan returned on 21 February.

This emergency situation was compounded by the drastic images in the world media from Bergamo, Italy. Around 4,500 people infected with the coronavirus died at that time, which was many times more than in similar periods in earlier years. From makeshift morgues in churches, coffins were transported by the army to distant crematoria, as the local ones were designed for a smaller number of the dead.

The SARS-CoV-2 pandemic also affected internal migrations. To counter the spread of the virus, arrivals and departures from towns in the province of Lodi in Lombardy and Vo in the province of Padua were restricted. Entry to these towns was guarded by police officers. Illegal departure from the area was made punishable by criminal penalties. The measures taken by the Italian authorities were unique in Europe.

International rail transport was also restricted. Connections between countries and Euroregions were suspended. After transit trains for citizens of the Baltic States and Ukraine were allowed to pass through the railway border crossings in the Visegrad countries, from mid-March 2020, only cargo trains passed through for several weeks. In the second half of March 2020, the Polish carrier PKP took measures that had a significant impact on internal migration. Out of the planned approximately 400 connections per day, as many as 281 were suspended, including all EIC (express intercity) connections. The remaining active connections were shortened and the number of carriages reduced. Similar decisions were taken by Czech (České Dráhy and GWTrain), Slovak (ZSSK) and Hungarian (MAV) carriers.

Restrictions on foreign and railway migration in the Visegrad Group area had different dimensions. In the first wave of the pandemic a state of emergency was declared in three V4 countries: Hungary, Slovakia and the Czech Republic; in Poland a state of emergency of an epidemic was declared. As a result – in varying rigour – people were forbidden to leave their flats and houses, and a curfew was imposed in some countries.

The situation of labour migrants during the SARS-CoV-2 pandemic deserves a separate discussion. Fears about the risk of coronavirus infection and the possible permanent closure of the EU's internal and external borders caused uncertainty for thousands of labour migrants. In a spontaneous and chaotic manner, thousands of them decided to return to their countries of origin in the EU. Similar were the reactions of labour migrants from post-Soviet countries – with the largest group appearing at the borders of EU Member States with Ukraine.

The consequence of the sudden outflow of workers from domestic labour markets was the reduction of agricultural works and production. However, the situation was exceptional in tourism and service activities. Hotels, guesthouses, restaurants, but also hairdressing salons – very often based on the work by labour migrants – were temporarily closed.

The pandemic also highlighted a huge change in attitudes towards cross-border workers. Restrictions on crossing borders have presented a large group of workers from Poland and the Czech Republic with the dilemma of staying in their country of origin or living in prepared and subsidised labour hotels abroad. Due to the high demand for cross-border workers, the authorities in the German federal states bordering Poland and the Czech Republic have decided to finance wage supplements and housing for the duration of the work. The governments of Brandenburg, Mecklenburg-Vorpommern and Sachsen have decided on such measures. The daily allowance of EUR 65 for an employee with a contract and an additional EUR 20 for a family member residing in Brandenburg and Mecklenburg-Vorpommern was a serious argument in stopping the outflow of labour to Poland. This was because it turned out that the allowance alone, amounting to as much as EUR 1,950 per month and an additional EUR 600 for a family member,[3] was well above the average wage in the foreign workers' countries of origin. The Sachsen authorities[4] provided lower allowances. They offered a daily allowance of EUR 40 and a family allowance of EUR 20, but the support was only aimed at those employed in the medical and long-term care sector. The programme benefited workers who, under the rules in force in Poland and the Czech Republic, would have been subject to a compulsory two-week quarantine in their countries of origin after working in Germany. However, due to uncertainty and fear of infection, many have decided not to work abroad.

A particular group of migrants are foreign students, who are also often service sector workers. In the period following the declaration of the pandemic, they found themselves in a difficult material situation due to not being able to work in tourism, services and as baby-sitters. However, the specificity of educational migrants in Central and Eastern Europe is that they come mainly from neighbouring countries. This is quite different from the situation of foreign students in the western EU Member States, where many thousands of students from other continents arrive every academic year.

The pandemic has also had an impact on the flow of people seeking international protection. Entry restrictions have forced thousands of potential asylum-seeking migrants to remain in their countries of origin. In January–October 2020, the number of new applicants[5] decreased by one-third compared to 2019 and amounted to 349 thousand people (Eurostat, 2021). Irregular border crossing also increased during the described period and amounted to 114 thousand persons. Flows between Turkey and Greece decreased significantly, while inflows to Malta, Italy and Spain increased. In the light of statistical data, a variation can be seen between the numbers of immigrants from different countries. In 2020, the number of immigrants from Syria, Tunisia and Algeria increased (Atlas of Migration, 2020, p. 467). During the attempts to enter the EU, 1,754 people died or went missing (Eurostat, 2021).

The number of people trying to obtain international protection in the Visegrad Group countries also decreased during the period in question. In Poland, the total number of applications for refugee status decreased by one-third. Only 1.5 thousand new applications were submitted – with a marked increase in the group of foreigners holding Belarusian citizenship. In the Czech Republic, 798 new applications for international protection[6] were submitted in 2020. The closure of transit routes is best illustrated by the fact that only 17 new applications were submitted in April 2020 (MVCR, 2021). Throughout 2020, 270 first applications were made in Slovakia and 80 in Hungary (Eurostat, 2021).

The several months that have passed since the announcement of the COVID-19 pandemic allow several key conclusions to be drawn. First and foremost, the restrictions on migration movements introduced in March 2020, then lifted over the vacation period and subsequently reintroduced, have become firmly embedded in the daily lives of societies in the EU Member States. While internal population movements have been restored, despite the rapidly increasing number of people vaccinated with one of the vaccines authorised for use within the EU, not all restrictions on cross-border movement have been lifted. An antigen or Polymerase Chain Reaction (PCR) test carried out 48 or 72 hours in advance is still required for entry into another country. If the traveller does not have a document confirming a negative result, he/she is directed to undergo a 10- or 14-day quarantine (e.g. in a designated COVID hotel).

Moreover, employers who have hitherto employed cross-border workers must take into account the unforeseen potential restrictions on the entry of this group of workers. Preventing the recruitment of cross-border workers will undoubtedly increase labour costs and the price of goods on offer. Employers taking in foreign workers have found themselves in a similar situation, and if they have provided services, they had to close down their businesses due to restrictions or have lost workers who have re-emigrated to their home countries.

Secondly, there is likely to be a reinforcement of the priority given to permanent migration, which, while it will raise labour costs and reduce the previous scale of free movement of workers, will signal increasing competition for foreign workers in the EU.

Thirdly, procedures related to the reception of migrants seeking asylum and possible relocation within the borders of the EU Member States (New Pact on Migration and Asylum, 2020) will be further streamlined. The solidarity approach and the efficient case management of people in critical life situations seeking international protection is probably the first step towards a comprehensive reform of the migration agenda in the EU – although much of the power over migration processes rests with Member State governments.

## 5.2 Labour market and unemployment during the pandemic

The increasing threat of the spread of the SARS-CoV-2 pandemic in late 2019 has affected the labour market. Both employers and employees found themselves in a new situation. It was necessary, on the one hand, to limit the possibility of direct contact of employees and, on the other hand, to maintain the continuity of the functioning of central and local government institutions, hospitals and medical clinics, educational institutions, companies and transport and the entire sphere of services.

Shortly after the identification of COVID-19 infected persons in the EU, a lockdown was declared in the Member States. This meant maximum restriction on the movement of people – an exception being, for example, leaving home for work when necessary.[7] This was a completely new situation for employers and employees. The solution was a kind of "transfer of work to the private sphere". It was based on the rapid development of teleworking and home office.[8]

Thanks to the development of IT services, it turned out to be possible to transfer a large part of one's duties away from one's current place of work in an office, school or company. State and private employers were equally affected, and the type of work performed became the main criterion deciding whether an employee should work from home. Digital versions of documents, widespread use of certified electronic signatures and the possibility to install and use the employer's professional IT programmes in the home environment resulted in most civil servants and office workers performing their duties at home. Manual workers did not have such an opportunity. Skilled and unskilled workers employed in manufacturing companies could stay at home if the employer decided to limit production. An example of such a restriction, which took place in March/April/May 2020, was in the automotive industry, where work is provided in individual factories and involves the simultaneous performance of certain activities by crew members. During the aforementioned period, work was suspended at, among others, Ford, Audi, BMW and VW factories across the EU. CNH Industrial closed factories in Italy. Similar action was taken at factories located in the Visegrad Group area – in Poland: Wielton, Dębica, MAN, Fiat Chrysler Automobiles, Opel and Michelin. In others, the work of particular departments (e.g. paint shops) was limited or production was simply reduced, as in the Hungarian and Polish Bridgestone plants.

The more than halved demand for new cars in the EU in March compared to February 2020 also resulted in decisions regarding employment levels. Employers who reported reduced sales of their products faced difficult decisions. In the Visegrad countries, these were not only companies from the automotive industry, but also, for example, the furniture industry – IKEA. Its representatives announced that they would lay off 150 workers as a result of the COVID-19 pandemic restrictions. In the small Polish town of Wielbark, with a population of less than 3,000, the decision by IKEA representatives has created a sense of social insecurity. In December 2020, Nidzica county, where Wielbark is situated, registered an unemployment rate of 7.1% (700 people), compared to 10.1% for Warmińsko-Mazurskie Region (51.5 thousand people) and 6.2% for Poland as a whole (GUS, 2021). It is worth underlining that together with the cities of Olsztyn and Elbląg as well as Gołdap county these were the counties that were affected the least by unemployment – in the remaining counties of the region unemployment reached two-digit figures.

It was in small towns, located at distances preventing daily, circular migration to work, that the COVID-19 pandemic had a very adverse effect on the labour market. As a consequence, those dealing with the situation in the labour market have found their monthly income reduced. Taking into account the low level of household savings in the Visegrad countries compared to the western part of the EU, the effect of loss of employment and monthly wages has become an increased risk of social marginalisation, including social exclusion.

The pandemic crisis has also affected travel and public transport services, as exemplified by the bankruptcy of the national Czechoslovak, and now Czech, carrier, Czech Airlines (ČSA), which was unable to generate revenue due to pandemic restrictions. On 10 March 2021, the carrier declared bankruptcy and laid off all its employees (430 people). Despite the bankruptcy, ČSA aircraft continue to operate on selected passenger routes, but financial problems and the threat to the future of the enterprise remained.

In order to protect the labour market and maintain the current level of employment, the governments of individual EU Member States decided to subsidise enterprises and the self-employed, who lost the possibility of earning income at the current level due to the forced closure of selected sectors of the economy. The aid was aimed mainly at the service sector: gastronomy (restaurants, cafes, bars), entertainment (theatres, cinemas, music bands and soloists), fitness and beauty industry (gyms, sports clubs, hairdressers and beauty salons).

On 13 March 2020, the German Ministers for Finance Olaf Scholz and for Economic Affairs and Energy Peter Altmaier presented the concept of a "protective shield" (*Schutzschild*) for employers and employees. First of all, the concept of shortened working hours (*Kurzarbeit*, KA) was included. This made it possible to shorten working hours, but also to reduce the remuneration received from the employer, with the difference in net remuneration being covered by the government. The idea was to make *Kurzarbeit* more widespread and to protect workers in times of pandemic. The programme also assumed that the costs of social insurance contributions for employees covered by the programme would be assumed by the Federal Employment Agency (*Bundesagentur für Arbeit*, BfA). Another measure planned in the German "protective shield" was the settlement of various taxes in favour of the payers, including even the suspension of enforcement proceedings until the end of 2020. The measures described above were complemented by support for measures enabling entrepreneurs to maintain liquidity and prevent payment bottlenecks and bankruptcies. Support was envisaged through low-cost loans and guarantees issued by the public credit bank (*Kreditanstalt für Wiederaufbau*, KfW) via commercial banks. Even further simplification of procedures is envisaged, so that – even if part of the risk is assumed – companies and employees are protected. In March 2020, the German authorities pledged EUR 460 billion for this purpose, with the possibility of increasing this amount by a further EUR 93 billion.

Measures to protect companies and workers have also been taken in the Visegrad countries. The Czech Republic provided the largest amount of assistance.[9] Under the established four programmes (Antivirus A Plus, Antivirus A, Antivirus B and Antivirus C), support is provided for entrepreneurs, including, inter alia: for the subsidisation of wages for employees of enterprises with a statutory ban on activities due to the COVID-19 pandemic and for the wages of quarantine employees.

Similar solutions have been adopted in Poland, where nine editions of the Anti-Crisis Shield programme[10] have already been launched since April 2020. Assistance was extended to both entrepreneurs and employees. Budget funds have been used to subsidise salaries of persons who have been covered by idle time pay or reduced working time. Support was available to employers who had lost income as a result of the reduction in business activity. Support was provided not only for large employers with a large number of employees but also for smaller entities (micro-entrepreneurs).

The Hungarian support measures for employers and employees had a specific dimension. In addition to the suspension of the payment of pension insurance premiums and a reduction of health insurance premiums, a ban on the termination of a lease or an increase in the lease fee was introduced for companies in the group affected by pandemic restrictions. Another unique solution was the rigid capping of the margin on consumer loans granted during the pandemic period at the central bank's base interest rate plus a maximum of 5%.

In Slovakia, the government also prepared a programme to support the economy, which was based primarily on the partial assumption by the state of employers' liabilities. As in other Visegrad countries, the focus was on labour market protection and support for the business sector at the same time.

The measures taken by the governments of the EU countries, including the Visegrad Group countries, were intended to support businesses and workers in the aftermath of the SARS-CoV-2 pandemic. The intention was to protect businesses as producers of GDP and as employers, and to protect the labour market, in the sense of preserving jobs so that they would be able to continue functioning normally in the post-COVID-19 pandemic period. The regulations that have been adopted have in fact made it possible for a number of companies to survive and, at the same time, have helped to maintain the level of consumption. This does not mean that the economies of the EU and Visegrad countries did not suffer as a result of COVID-19. Detailed information in this regard is provided by the *Spring 2021 Economic Forecast: Rolling up sleeves*, which shows that GDP calculated for the EU Member States as a whole decreased by 6.1%. Significant above-average GDP declines were recorded in Spain (–10.8%), France (–8.1%), Italy (–8.9%), Greece (–8.2%) and Croatia (–8%). In contrast, the lowest GDP declines were recorded in Luxembourg (–1.3%) and Lithuania (–0.9%); still low, but already higher GDP decline was also registered in Poland and Denmark (–2.7%), Sweden and Finland (–2.8%) and Estonia (–2.9%). The European Commission's 2021 data shows that Poland's economy was the least affected by the pandemic, followed by Slovakia and Hungary, and the Czech Republic was affected the worst. The economic situation of the Visegrad Group countries is conditioned by a number of factors – including the structure of enterprises and the specificity of the products they manufacture. The forecasts presented for 2021 show that the GDP of Hungary and Slovakia will recover faster than the GDP of Poland and the Czech Republic.[11]

The effectiveness of the solutions taken by the authorities of the Visegrad Group countries can also be measured by taking into account the unemployment rate. Over the period 2020-2021, the unemployment rate increased in the EU Member States from 7.1% to 7.6%, including in the euro zone from 7.8% to 8.4%. The highest increases in the unemployment rate were recorded in Ireland (from 5.7% to 10.7%), Belgium (from 5.6% to 6.7%), Estonia (from 6.8% to 7.9%) and the Czech Republic (from 2.6% to 3.8%). In several countries the unemployment rate remained unchanged (Greece, Malta, Slovenia, Hungary) and even decreased in a few (Cyprus, Lithuania, Austria, Portugal, Bulgaria, Denmark, Croatia, Sweden).

Statistics presented by the European Commission show that in different EU Member States, the impact of the pandemic on the economic situation varied. The huge financial resources allocated from the budgets of the Member States undoubtedly had a positive impact on the situation of businesses and enterprises and on workers, enabling them to survive during the period of greatest restrictions – services in particular.

## 5.3 Climate policy in the pandemic period

The pandemic period has had a negative impact on countries' climate policies. For example, the planned December 2020 summit in Glasgow (COP26) was cancelled due to the COVID-19 pandemic. In the background of climate policy considerations is also the question of overcoming possible economic consequences after the COVID-19 pandemic and supporting the economic recovery process. The coincidence of the occurrence of the COVID-19 pandemic and climate policy measures is a very negative development for overcoming the effects of the pandemic.

This important issue has become increasingly entrenched in public consciousness systematically since the 1970s and the emergence of the Club of Rome's Project analyses of the natural resources of planet earth (Meadows et al., 1972). The establishment of the Intergovernmental Panel on Climate Change (IPCC), and later two international institutions, the United Nations Environment Programme (UNEP) and the World Meteorological Organisation (WMO), was important in broadening environmental awareness. It was the 1990 IPCC report that described the problem of the greenhouse effect, which is accelerated by human activity (Houghton et al., 1990, p. VII). The report's conclusions then formed the basis for the United Nations Framework Convention on Climate Change (UNFCCC), which referred to limiting greenhouse gas emissions. Climate issues were later discussed at the 1992 United Nations Conference on Environment and Development in Rio de Janeiro and were reflected in the international treaty signed in December 1997 in Kyoto.

Of key importance for the EU Member States was the commitment adopted at the Paris Climate Conference (COP21) in December 2015, which is the first universal and legally binding climate agreement (Paris Agreement, 2015). It was joined by almost 190 countries, including the

European Union and its Member States.[12] Importantly, the Paris Agreement emphasises the role of regions, local authorities, civil society, the private sector and city authorities. It seems that the document is extremely accurate in identifying those actors who can most effectively contribute to limiting the increase in global temperature and greenhouse gas emissions.

Observing the European Union's actions in the area of combating climate change, it can be stated that it is an international leader in positive changes.[13]

The main objective of the EU's climate policy – expressed in the Introduction to the European Green Deal – is to become the first climate-neutral continent (Der europäische Grüne Deal, 2019, p. 1). In order to achieve these goals, more efficient energy use and an increase in the use of renewable energies have been assumed.

During the COVID-19 pandemic, in December 2020, the European Commission presented the 2030 Roadmap, in which the EU Member States were committed to a significant reduction of net greenhouse gas emissions in the EU by 2030 (by at least 40% compared to 1990 levels[14]), the use of minimum 32% of energy from renewable sources and to improve energy efficiency (32.5%).

The EU Member States have long been taking measures to reduce greenhouse gas emissions and make significantly more efficient use of natural resources. Climate-protection-oriented NGOs, as well as individual representatives of particular communities, are playing a huge role. A good example of such commitment is the minor Greta Thunberg from Sweden, who, speaking in August 2018 on behalf of the younger generation, drew attention to the progressive, irreversible climate change. Her participation in the Katowice Climate Summit (COP24) in 2018 underlined the importance of the Youth Climate Strike.

In particular, the popularisation of climate-conscious attitudes among children and young people suffered due to the COVID-19 pandemic. This was linked to the suspension or reduction of direct, stationary education organised in school facilities.

Climate policy issues are of particular importance in the Visegrad countries. This is due to the unfavourable structure of the energy balance in these countries, which is the result of the energy sector being based on non-renewable energy sources or on nuclear energy from power stations built using energy-intensive technology developed in the USSR. Renewable energy sources need to be developed, but this is associated with large financial outlays – for example, for the development of wind farms. Thanks to government subsidies and growing climate awareness, the area of wind farms and photovoltaic panels is increasing.

Among the Visegrad countries, the greatest changes in the structure of the energy balance must take place in Poland, where, despite the projects announced back in the 1980s before the fall of communism, no nuclear power plant has been built yet and, as a result, a significant proportion of energy is obtained from non-renewable sources. In the period of the pandemic in Poland – despite the historic drop in the level of energy produced from hard coal and lignite, energy production from these sources has amounted to as much as 70%, with as little as 18% of energy being produced from renewable energy sources (wind, sun), 10% as a result of gas combustion and the remaining 2% of energy being imported. The change in the balance structure is evidenced by the fact that compared to 2019 the production of energy from renewable sources has increased by 10% and from gas by 20%, and, significantly, the use of energy from coal has decreased by more than 10% (Informacja, 2021, p. 15).

In other Visegrad countries the energy balance looks much more optimistic, for example, in Hungary only 9% of energy is obtained from coal, 29% from oil and 32% from natural gas, while 16% of energy is obtained from nuclear power plants (Egedy et al., 2020, p. 143). As already mentioned, in Hungary, Slovakia and the Czech Republic a total of six nuclear power plants[15] are in operation and there are plans to expand this energy sector precisely in order to reduce emissions of climate-harming substances. The construction of a nuclear power station is also planned in Poland, although this process is very much behind schedule due to the strong influence of the coal lobby. There are 26 active mines in Poland and a further 16 are in the process of decommissioning, with a total of 138,000 people employed in the mining sector.[16] Employment levels and stakeholder organisation are a brake on the path to change.

The COVID-19 pandemic has come at a critical time for climate policy consolidation in the EU and Visegrad countries. The need for change is virtually unquestioned, but it is coupled unfavourably with possible adverse changes in restoring the economy to its pre-pandemic state. This is basically the only problem.

## 5.4 Solving social problems (crime, loneliness of the elderly, cultural-psychological problems) in the period of the pandemic

The period of the COVID-19 pandemic has witnessed a change in the priorities of the state's social policy, limited infrastructural and human resources, and partly also financial resources, directed at activities aimed at protecting the population from the SARS-CoV-2 virus, causing marginalisation of activities enabling the counteraction of social problems, including crime prevention, loneliness of the elderly and prevention of cultural-psychological problems.

Leaders of countries of the prosperous North – including the EU Member States – faced a difficult ethical choice. It had to be decided which measures to prioritise. Firstly, it was judged that, above all, the proliferation of the virus needed to be restrained. Secondly, it was recognised that COVID-19-infected persons require intensive care and separate, self-contained treatment sites. These decisions resulted in the involvement of law enforcement services in activities of an exceptional nature, such as checking the places where people under isolation or quarantine stay, commercial establishments, restaurants or service places. Statistical data show a change in the structure of crimes committed. There has been a significant decrease in the number of fights, thefts and robberies, while there has been a significant increase in the number of car thefts, murders and economic crimes.

In light of the above, it can be seen that the number of offences involving direct contact between the perpetrator and the victim, as well as the movement of perpetrators, has decreased. Increased crime statistics, in turn, involve offences committed as a result of cohabitation, growing demand for individual means of transport and online document circulation on an unprecedented scale (Kriminalita dle TSK, 2020; KSH, 2020).

This was facilitated by the aforementioned involvement of law enforcement services in the support of medical personnel, as well as the late reporting of incidents, for example, car thefts due to prolonged stay at home. For many criminals, the fact that direct contact between businesses or with authorities was reduced provided an excellent opportunity for abuse. They applied for funding from anti-crisis programmes, avoided paying tax obligations or carried out fraudulent business transactions. At the same time, law enforcement officers (police, civil guards, municipal guards) during the pandemic also expected their safety to be taken into account and, as far as possible, not to be exposed to the risk of infection. Some officers were forced to exercise their right to remain at home to look after underage children.

Prosecution of all crimes committed during the COVID-19 pandemic will only become possible once officers and civilian law enforcement personnel are fully vaccinated. Given the delay in reporting, the obliteration of traces of crimes and the running time of the statute of limitations, it can be assumed that some perpetrators of criminal acts will nevertheless escape punishment. In light of the actions taken by the governments of the Visegrad Group countries, it can be concluded that the above was considered a lesser social problem than the widespread threat to life caused by the SARS-CoV-2 virus.

A similar approach was adopted for problems related to the care of the elderly. Although medical studies showed that it is people in the post-productive age group who are more vulnerable to the undesirable effects of the virus (more severe course of the disease, higher mortality rate), it is this group against which the actions of medical and social services have proved to be the least effective. Above all, people in communal care homes have been massively infected. It is presumed that they were infected by medical staff working in hospitals with COVID-19 wards and at the same time providing medical advice to seniors in nursing homes.

Another traumatic experience for healthy and independent elderly people was the feeling of loneliness, both during confinement in flats and in the last moments of life in isolated COVID wards set up in temporary halls or tents. In the Visegrad countries, this situation was also due to mass post-accession migration, which resulted in people of mobile working age going abroad and leaving their parents behind in their country of origin. Difficulties in crossing borders resulted in a situation in which older people relied solely on themselves, social services and neighbours. It should be stressed that while in rural areas there were neighbourhood and family ties established over generations, and older people could count on the help of people they knew, in metropolitan cities, especially in city centres, where temporary accommodation was widespread and there was a high risk of infection (lift, shop, pharmacy, doctor's surgery), older people felt helpless in the initial phase of lockdown. During this period, to make things easier for them, "senior citizens' hours" were introduced, during which only older people were served in shops. The city's social services (care workers, social workers) took a special interest in providing for the elderly. A network of volunteers – young people – was organised to respond to the needs of senior citizens: they collected lists of necessary products and purchased and delivered them to the indicated address. National guard officers, police officers and social workers also performed a similar function. They organised the delivery of food but also, in the case of necessary medical appointments, took senior citizens to clinics and health centres.

A major and unforeseen problem for the elderly, however, has been the reduction of medical services provided in outpatient clinics and the postponement of planned surgeries until the number of COVID-19-caused illnesses declines. In Poland, the likely result of this reduction has been a sharp increase in the recorded number of deaths to 485,000 – 67,000 more than in 2019 (Informacja o zgonach, 2021, p. 2). The peak in deaths of older people occurred in November 2020, when there was a 106% increase compared to 2019 (Information on deaths, p. 3). Undoubtedly, this exceptionally high number of deaths was due to the severity of COVID-19 infection and coincided with an increase in the number of illnesses, but also a kind of "freezing" of medical services for people with chronic illnesses and the psychological impact of residential isolation.

The feeling of loneliness among the elderly was intensified by reduced participation in family and religious celebrations. With the pandemic, restrictions were placed on the number of people attending: church services, religious festivals, weddings and funerals. Compared to other Visegrad countries, seniors in Poland have felt this form of isolation the most. Sharing holidays or attending a holy mass on Sunday is a Polish tradition that had never before been violated on such a scale.

The feeling of insecurity and isolation – especially among socially and professionally active people living alone and away from relatives – caused an increase in undesirable cultural and psychological behaviour. After an initial stage of euphoria and satisfaction with staying at home (while receiving the remuneration for work), there came a second stage which gave rise to resentment against being forced to stay at home and reinforced the need to return to the previous lifestyle, to meet with friends and to return to professional life. It was then that attempts were made to circumvent the restrictions. In the EU Member States, young people sought ways to bypass the rules. Lending a pet became a symbol of such behaviour – walking the dog was a legal reason for leaving one's home.

Similar reactions arose in relation to the banning of gyms, fitness clubs and amateur sports clubs. Discussions in online forums and social networks questioned the advisability of this ban, pointing out that physical culture promotes better fitness and health. Faced with the further closure of the "fitness industry", some clubs started to operate illegally.[17]

Apart from seniors, the period of isolation and quarantine was particularly badly endured by children and young people. The youngest, accustomed to physical activity and regular meetings with their peers, were forced overnight to spend many hours in front of computer screens. Several days after the closure of primary schools in the Visegrad countries, education was organised in remote form, using modern technologies to conduct online lessons and send files with educational materials and videos. This new form did not work well for children in primary education.

The advisability of holding online lessons for many hours with this group of pupils was very often criticised by parents observing such teaching attempts and by psychologists who pointed to psychological and physical conditions which prevented effective learning in this form. The youngest children had problems with logging on to some classes, remembering the dates of lessons and, finally, concentrating on the subject of the class. Another difficulty was access to internet transmissions of varying quality, which mainly affected children living outside cities.

Forced stays in homes, limited contact with peers and friends, and exclusion from work have had a negative impact on the mental health of citizens in the EU Member States. The number of psychological consultations has increased. On the basis of data from the Polish Social Insurance Institution, the number of sick leaves for employees on account of depression has risen by as much as 19%. In 2020, mental and behavioural disorders accounted for as much as 10.8% of total sick leave (Komunikat ZUS, 2021).

Actions such as concerts for other residents performed on balconies, changes in lighting and even a dance performed by young Polish police officers for children isolated at home, spontaneously organised at the beginning of the COVID-19 pandemic by residents of large housing estates, were not able to sufficiently alleviate the dysfunction associated with forced separation from neighbours, relatives or friends. Aggressive behaviour of people who were reminded on the streets, in shops and on public transport to cover their noses and mouths also turned out to be a specific symptom of the tensions. The Visegrad countries' police forces intervened in such cases, but these incidents were by no means incidental.

The actual effects of the change in priorities of state institutions in counteracting important social problems will only be properly assessed in the long term. Contrary to critical voices emphasising restrictiveness and limitation of civil liberties, it should be assumed that decision-makers acted in a reactive manner, but the situation was unprecedented, and the risk to the safety and lives of citizens too high to hesitate.

Another unresolved question is to what extent the consequences of the pandemic described above will affect the further functioning of societies:

interpersonal contacts, the level of mutual trust, and techniques for resolving disputes and conflicts among social groups. It can definitely be stated that the discussed change of social policy priorities in the EU countries – including the Visegrad Group – has become an important experience for entire societies, the unforeseen consequence of which may be closer cooperation and deeper integration in the future.

The SARS-CoV-2 pandemic was a surprising and profound experience for world leaders. The ways and extent of countering the impact varied considerably. The widest protection of the population and economy was proposed in the countries of the prosperous North. Leaders of the EU countries managed to completely change the social and economic lifestyles of their countries for several months during the first three waves of the pandemic.

Due to the uniqueness of the situation, decisions concerning limiting social contacts, building temporary hospitals, changing forms of providing work and organising education, as well as limiting medical services for chronic diseases or restricting migration flows, were spontaneous and reactive. In assessing the actions of the Visegrad countries, it is important to point to the specificity of the post-communist societies, which have proved to be more disciplined. The reason for this, however, is not necessarily the experience of living under a totalitarian regime in the older generations, but the much smaller material resources of the state and society, and thus the greater risk of having to bear the consequences of imprudent actions themselves.

The decision by the EU representatives to purchase and dispose of vaccine preparations collectively should also be regarded as excellent. Thanks to this decision, it was possible to provide individual countries with vaccines efficiently and to avoid international conflicts as a result of competition among manufacturers.

Several months after the end of the third wave of the pandemic, it is difficult to assess which country from the EU or Visegrad Group performed best. It is impossible to adopt an objective criterion, as the population levels in these countries differ, for example, it is difficult to compare the actions of the Finnish authorities, where the population is low, with those of the German or French authorities, where agglomerations such as Paris or the Ruhr region are located. However, the pandemic has made the leaders of the Visegrad countries aware that perhaps a shift in the funding stream from social benefits to salaries for medical staff should be considered. This issue came up very clearly in the Czech Republic and Poland, where there were shortages of medical staff. In the Czech Republic, this has even led to a wider discussion in relation to the admission of Czech patients by German hospitals.

It can be assumed that the restrictions on migration processes during the pandemic will change the previous rules on population flows. Freedom and spontaneity in the face of an epidemic threat must be limited and included in a new system of migration management – especially those with an external (transcontinental) dimension.

The labour market is also likely to change by shifting more of the actual cost of providing labour to the worker in the remote work system. Employers who have implemented the expansion of this form of work will benefit from the opportunity to reduce the costs of providing workspace. Issues related to the depreciation of the working environment, equipment and the responsibility for the health of the employee working from home will probably be the subject of work of the legislative bodies in the near future.

The shutting down of street lighting in Krakow may be regarded as a peculiar symbol of the pandemic. Such a situation has not occurred since the blackout organised during the Second World War. We can only hope that the medium- and long-term effects of the pandemic will be less significant than those caused by warfare.

## Notes

1 For example, in the first days of March 2020 as many as two-thirds of rail connections were cancelled in Poland.
2 Organised by the Polish government in cooperation with the Polish carrier PLL Lot, the action did not include other citizens of the EU countries.
3 The average wage of a worker in Poland was EUR 1150, in Hungary EUR 1140, in Slovakia EUR 1099, in the Czech Republic EUR 1,326 (Eurostat, 2021).
4 According to estimates, there were about 10,000 cross-border workers from Poland employed in Sachsen.
5 These are persons making applications on arrival in the territory of one of the EU Member States whose applications have not previously been examined.
6 In addition, 366 further (repeat) applications were received.
7 Movement for essential living needs – including walking pets – was also permitted. Curfews were introduced in some EU Member States, restricting private movement at night.
8 Teleworking is a form of work regulated by the Labor Codex, the official rules of remote work were introduced by the so-called Covid Act of March 2020. The main difference is that the employee's consent to this form of work is not required in the case of remote work (as a result, the employee can be dismissed).
9 In the first wave of the COVID-19 pandemic it was about 18% of the Czech Republic's GDP (approx. EUR 36 billion).
10 The first edition of the Anti-Crisis Shield was adopted on 1 April 2020, the next on 17 April 2020; the programmes are numbered from 1.0 to 9.0.
11 https://ec.europa.eu/info/business-economy-euro/economic-performance-and-forecasts/economic-forecasts/spring-2021-economic-forecast-rolling-sleeves_en
12 The EU ratified the agreement on 5 October 2016; it entered into force on 4 November 2016. The agreement had to be ratified by at least 55 countries responsible for a minimum of 55% of global greenhouse gas emissions.
13 The EU has played a significant role in negotiating the Paris Agreement.
14 An update is being prepared that includes a 55% reduction in emissions compared to 1990.
15 Of which: 3 in the Czech Republic, 2 in Hungary and 1 in Slovakia.
16 https://ibs.org.pl/app/uploads/2020/09/IBS_Research_Report_01_2020.pdf
17 Restaurants operated in a similar way during the ban; the windows on the street side of the restaurant were sealed tightly and only customers who made an arrangement were served.

# References

Atlas of Migration (2020). *Atlas of Migration.* European Commission, Joint Research Centre, Luxembourg.

Der europäische Grüne Deal (2019). *Der europäische Grüne Deal.* Mitteilung der Kommission, Europaeische Kommission, Brüssel, den 11.12.2019, COM(2019) 640 final

Dudek, D., Husak, Z., Kowalski, G., & Lis, W. (2013). *Konstytucyjny system organów państwa.* C.H. Beck.

Egedy A., Gyurik, L., Ulbert, Z., & Rado, A. (2020). CFD modeling and environmental assessment of a VOC removal silo. *International Journal of Environmental Science and Technology,* 18(5), pp. 141–150. DOI: 10.1007/s13762-020-02833-7

Eurostat (2021). *Five main citizenships of first-time asylum applicants (non-EU citizens).* Available from: https://ec.europa.eu/eurostat/statistics-explained/images/a/a1/Table_1_Five_main_citizenships_of_first-time_asylum_applicants_%28non-EU_citizens%29%2C_2020_%28number%2C_rounded_figures%29_v2.png

GUS (2021). *Informacja o liczbie bezrobotnych zarejestrowanych oraz stopa bezrobocia według statystycznego podziału kraju (rewizja NUTS 2016) oraz administracyjnego podziału terytorialnego kraju (TERYT).* Stan w końcu grudnia 2020 r.[xlsx]

Houghton, J.T., Jenkins, G.J., & Ephraums, J.J. (Eds.) (1990). *Climate Change. The IPCC Scientific Assessment.* Cambridge University Press.

Informacja (2021). Informacja statystyczna o energii elektrycznej. *Biuletyn miesięczny,* styczeń 2021, No. 1 (325), Agencja Rynku Energii SA.

Informacja o zgonach (2021). *Informacja o zgonach w Polsce w 2020 roku* (luty 2021). Departament Analiz i Strategii, Ministerstwo Zdrowia.

Komunikat ZUS (2021). Komunikat ZUS. Available from: https://www.zus.pl/o-zus/aktualnosci/-/publisher/aktualnosc/1/w-2020-r_-najwiecej-zwolnien-lekarskich-wystawiono-w-marcu-i-pazdzierniku/3968073

Kriminalita dle TSK (2020). Kriminalita dle TSK – podrobná sestava O POČTECH SKUTKŮ A ŠKODÁCH na org. článku ČESKÁ REPUBLIKA, období 1.1. – 31.12.2020, Statistické přehledy kriminality za rok 2020, Policie České republiky

KSH (2020). Hungarian Central Statistical Office (KSH) 2021, 11.1.2.1. Registered crimes by county and region.

Meadows, D., Meadows, D., Randers, J., & Behrens III, W. (1972). *The Limits to Growth: A report for the Club of Rome's Project on the Predicament of Mankind.* Universe Books.

MVCR (2021). *Počty žádostí o mezinárodní ochranu v jednotlivých měsících roku 2020.* Available from: https://www.mvcr.cz/migrace/docDetail.aspx?docid=22238075&doctype=ART

New Pact on Migration and Asylum (2020). *New Pact on Migration and Asylum.* September 2020, European Commission.

Paris Agreement (2015). *Paris Agreement 2015.* United Nations.

# 6   State and society in times of a pandemic

*Ewa Maria Marciniak and Marcin Tobiasz*

## 6.1  Politicians and society in the face of a crisis – an attempt at political analysis

The beginning of the 1990s was a time of dreams about the end of history and a post-political era in the history of mankind. "Politics", however, reminded us of itself as early as 2008 during the economic crisis, which "bred a deep distrust of business elites and the casino capitalism that, *writ large*, almost destroyed the world financial order" (Krastew & Holmes, 2020, p. 27). However, the economic crisis mentioned by the cited authors led to much more serious political consequences. The myth of liberal democracy collapsed and the process of erosion of trust in the Western state as a model for humanity began. Time slowly erased in the collective memory the dark sides of non-liberalism, and the weakening position of the West in the world awakened questions about the universality of the model and its non-alternativeness.

> The lack of a plausible alternative to liberal democracy became a stimulus to revolt because, at some elemental level, "human beings need choice, even just the illusion of it". Populists are rebelling not only against a specific (liberal) type of politics but also as against the replacement of communist orthodoxy by liberal orthodoxy. The message of insurgent movements on both the left and the right, in effect, is that a take-it-or-leave-it approach is wrong and that things can be different, as well as more familiar and more authentic.
>
> (Krastew & Holmes, 2020, p. 6)

The democracies of Central and Eastern Europe, lauded for their transformation, have changed

> into conspiracy-minded majoritarian regimes where the political opposition was demonised, non-government media, civil society and independent courts were denuded of their influence, and sovereignty was defined as the leadership's determination to resist any and all pressure to conform to Western ideals of political pluralism,

DOI: 10.4324/9781003353812-7

government transparency and tolerance for strangers, dissidents and minorities.

(Krastew & Holmes, 2020, p. 25)

While in the early years of the political transition in Central and Eastern Europe liberalism was associated with the ideals of opportunity for everyone, freedom of movement and travel, allowing difference of opinion, access to justice and government responsiveness to the demands of society, after 2010 growing social inequalities, pervasive corruption and morally arbitrary redistribution of public property into the hands of a small, privileged group made it a godsend that failed.

The pandemic caused by the SARS-CoV-2 coronavirus has placed governments and societies around the world in a very different, new and, above all, crisis political situation. How individual governments dealt with this challenge depended not only on organisational efficiency but also on their ability to communicate with the public, mutual perception of threats and understanding of the nature of state action and social responses. The uncertainty resulting from the new situation could lead to questioning the decisions of those in power, and even to actively demonstrating opposition to them. Maintaining social peace as a result of mutual understanding thus became a very important objective for decision-makers. The liberal perception of politics, which has been dominating not only in Europe but also worldwide since the 1990s, is still rooted in the theory of rational choice and its basic assumption, according to which everyone, including politicians, is guided in their actions by rational self-interest, aiming at its maximisation. Thus, measures to counter the spread of a pandemic and its effects have become at least controversial. This paradigm prepared a wide ground for the de-politicisation of the democratic state model itself, which ceased to be perceived as an effective system of representation of social interests, as it gradually placed the fate of citizens in the hands of experts and technocrats rather than elected representatives (Hay, 2007). Professionals, on the other hand, tend to treat citizens more as passive observers who need to be mobilised when necessary. This problem affects the entire political system, including, for example, NGOs, which have ceased to rely on mass membership and have begun to rely on professional campaign organisers. Citizens have begun to be treated as an audience that is usually addressed through media campaigns and expected at most to occasionally sign a letter or participate in an organised demonstration. There is no deep, analytical message, only simple messages. What is required is, at most, the occasional involvement of a wider group of citizens in an organised "event" such as a protest or a political rally. Such a shallow experience has a marginal effect and rather perpetuates the conviction that there is no real influence on political decisions. It is more a lifestyle, a form of public statement than a serious, conscious engagement in political debate. Political participation thus becomes ephemeral, sporadic and shallow. Just expressing an opinion is only the beginning, because politics is not only the ability to express one's views but also the art of listening to others and making collective decisions. It is a process of finding collective solutions to specific problems among different social groups with often divergent or even contradictory interests, values and views, and requires a difficult allocation of scarce resources that is acceptable to all. Politics at the level of large, interconnected and diverse societies is a challenge. It should reflect our collective will, which is not easily grasped and, above all, changes over time and needs to be subordinated as it will already be expressed at the level of a concrete decision. It is a very demanding but also the most edifying human experience requiring going beyond self-interest (Hay & Stoker, 2009, pp. 231–234). Subordinated to economically understood rationality, politics has become a kind of puzzle or a simple mathematical equation with only one correct solution, which just has to be discovered. It is also often portrayed as an arena of sport competition where there can only be one winner, rather than a complex decision-making process that allows for different viewpoints and expectations to be taken into account.

A pandemic is not only a new situation and one that requires unconventional measures but also a crisis. This means that it is associated with more or less violent disorders, leading to the destabilisation of some spheres of social life. Elements of the situation, which so far have been characterised by relative congruence, order and functionality, are to some extent disrupted, leading to a crisis. The pandemic required, as Boin and co-authors point out in their article, learning (Boin et al., 2020) – learning in terms of how decision-makers responded, how political leaders regained control of the situation, and new social responses. "Normal modes of policymaking had to be abandoned, as conventional toolkits and contingency plans proved ineffective" (Boin et al., 2020).

Under conditions of uncertainty, ignorance and lack of clarity about the possible outcomes of the crisis, it becomes particularly important for policymakers to work with the public. The nature and quality of these mutual relations determine the effects of actions taken, i.e. de facto effectiveness in dealing with a completely new and crisis situation, which was the COVID-19 pandemic. An extremely important role in building these relations is played by the media, which, on the one hand, are only a carrier of information, and on the other hand, are also its creators and active political actors. Unfortunately, the 24-hour media and social media, in their pursuit of audiences and profit, are reducing the quality of the information they provide and are allowing a flood of fake news, which, especially during the pandemic, has become downright dangerous, because the mass consumer does not have the contextual knowledge needed to verify the presented content. As a result, citizens receive a simplified and sensationalised picture of current politics – highlighting its negative features, as these are more sought after (Karwat, 2012).

Focusing on the negative side of politicians' activities fosters widespread scepticism towards politics in general and governments' actions in combating pandemics. The solitary following of events and actions taken via social media accompanied by the occasional like or comment cannot replace face-to-face interactions and public debate. Weighing alternatives has been devalued as a democratic benchmark in favour of the practice of seeking widespread, often tacit approval. The generally declining level of news coverage, in a situation where the media has become the main source of information on COVID-19, results in a deformed and simplified message against the actual complexity of the problem. The emotionally driven media spread a culture of contempt, hatred and fear, and journalists often gain their social accreditation in opposition to politicians, portraying them in a negative light, as fraudsters who need to be constantly monitored, watched and exposed. In such conditions democracy becomes its own caricature. The social engineering of fear in the hands of skilful politicians is an excellent technology for managing the masses, making it possible to avoid uncomfortable and time-consuming discussions under the guise of preserving the democratic façade. It is enough to create a sense of threat and to point to only the right and easy-to-implement solution. Such a technique polarises and allows "our" solution to be presented as the natural opposition to the undesirable state of affairs. This provides an ideal breeding ground for all sorts of populism, and during a pandemic it became a tool for introducing political changes convenient to those in power under the pretext of combating the pandemic.

The role of the media in a pandemic requires a broader analysis. The perception of risks by decision-makers and the public may be fundamentally different, but the cooperation of those in power with the media in such a system becomes crucial during a pandemic to reduce uncertainty in society. Thus, it can be hypothesised that the role of the media in times of pandemics increases, as they can become an effective tool in the hands of those in power, thanks to which their decisions, for example, on the management of restrictions, become understandable to citizens. A specific measure of the effects of communication between the rulers and society is the results of surveys conducted by opinion poll centres. This is because polls reflect the degree of comprehensibility of the decisions of those in power and the degree of support or negation for the adopted solutions. Additionally, it may be assumed that in a crisis situation the communication of public-opinion leaders with the public becomes particularly important. This means not only active politicians but also new actors in public communication.

If one assumes that the perception of threats by those in power and society is conditioned by a reciprocal relationship, it is a kind of feedback. This feedback stems from the fact that the type and scale of actions taken by policymakers are, on the one hand, the result of an analysis of public mood and expectations, while on the other hand, the public may assess the risks resulting from the pandemic as small or large through the prism of the size or spectacularism of actions taken by the government. Therefore, we are dealing here with two types of actions: *proactive actions* – imposing certain solutions and formal and legal regulations, including restrictions, on society – and *reactive actions*, which result from the diagnosis of the importance of social behaviour (e.g. gathering without observing the sanitary regime) and the survey of public moods, which is the result of analyses of experts and advisory bodies. Either way, the perception of risks by decision-makers and the public is mutually conditioned in terms of the forms and content of action. Public opinion polls reflect these two types of government action; they permeate each other and are also mutually determined. The effect of these actions can be described through the prism of two levels of coherence: *sequential* (actions staggered over time and messages about them) and *simultaneous* (e.g. actions/restrictions at the same time, differentiated towards different actors). Sequential coherence refers to the degree of coherence vs. incoherence of decisions during COVID-19 made in a specific sequence of time.[1] Simultaneous coherence – closure of forests, shopping malls, active churches and large home improvement stores, clubs and discos (March 2020 in Poland) – is an example of a low degree of coherence, or essentially simultaneous incoherence. This lack of logical connection in the decisions of those in power was not conducive to reaching a consensus on the interpretation of the COVID-19 threat.[2]

The ontological openness of the analysed processes makes it difficult to conclude whether and to what extent the pandemic will change the perception of policy and organisation of the state that has prevailed since the 1990s. Will it be possible to revitalise the public sphere and restore the recently forgotten meaning of the term *politics* as the ability to act in a situation of real collective or social choice? This means that politics should be everywhere, where we are not dealing with the determination of our fate but with its co-shaping by citizens. Matters over which we have no influence as citizens thus belong to the realm of non-politics. Politicisation, then, means nothing less than including an issue in the process of deliberation, decision-making and action in the public sphere. De-politicisation, on the other hand, is the opposite process, i.e. exclusion of issues from the public debate and depriving citizens of the possibility of real decision-making and elections (Hay & Stoker, 2009, pp. 67–81).

Politicisation in a broad sense means revealing and questioning what is taken for granted and without alternative. The strategy of de-politicisation entails fatalism and necessity, which limits the human capacity to act, choose and change the existing world (Jenkins, 2011, pp. 159–160). It leads to the presentation of certain orders as ultimately justified, for example scientifically or morally, and thus unquestionable. Thus, particularism is presented as a negation of neutrality and impartiality, and politics as a game devoid of any rules, a space for manipulation. The world outlined in opposition is presented as free of political interests, i.e. of particularism. The result is a de-politicisation of difference and the replacement of politics with administration. What emerges is a top-down defined set of issues and problems that cannot be the subject of social choices. The depoliticising practices themselves are presented not as a destruction of diversity, a reduction of choice and available alternatives, but as a liberation from socially destructive particularisms. In this context, politicisation means opposing domination, where power relations limit the activity that would mean the possibility of the formulation and existence of a political alternative.

Politics, which has an inherently complex character, should be treated as a creative, undetermined process during which participants appeal to different values and have at least the potential to question the actions taken by those in power and even to change the existing order. Without a real possibility of modifying the existing social order, or even a belief in such a possibility, there can be no politics. Wherever we influence others through action there is politics. However, social and governmental strategies for recognising or denying the possibility of human will can differ fundamentally, as it became vividly apparent during the pandemic caused by the SARS-CoV-2 coronavirus.

## 6.2 Politics in times of a pandemic and clarification of social attitudes as a result of government activity in V4 countries: Poland in comparison with the Czech Republic, Slovakia and Hungary

The beginning of 2020 was a time of political recognition and definition of threats related to the pandemic and designing legal regulations. These took the form of laws and executive acts which introduced restrictions consisting, in general, in the closure of cultural and sports facilities, schools and universities, workplaces, catering facilities and parks. Assemblies were banned, and even leaving places of residence was forbidden. The introduced restrictions and the narratives used by governments on the COVID-19 pandemic were reflected in public opinion surveys. These surveys initially focused on the type and strength of response to the pandemic. Opinion poll centres provided a variety of data showing public opinions on the decisions made and their adequacy to the situation. It should be noted that in different countries the intensity of social research varies, as does the number of centres studying public opinion. Therefore, their results will not always be comparable. The decisions of governments referred to various spheres of social life: education, transport, economy, assemblies, sports and cultural events, and were generally understood and accepted. An example of such a diagnosis is the study carried out in Poland by Krystyna Skarżyńska for the Batory Foundation (Maj & Skarżyńska, 2020).

In light of the findings of the above-mentioned study, in the initial period of the pandemic, strict adherence to the epidemic safety recommendations provided by the Polish authorities was accepted by 82.4% of respondents, while in the survey conducted again – 73.4% expressed their acceptance of these decisions. However, the acceptance of the government's actions was accompanied by negative emotions, among which the author includes shock and fear. This may be related to the fact that media coverage of dramas and misfortunes – especially in Lombardy, Italy – may have intensified these emotions to a large extent. In addition, there was also concern about the state of one's own health and that of one's loved ones, followed by gradually increasing concern about the efficiency of the health service and the economy. In all V4 countries, research confirms that fear for one's own health and that of loved ones, concern about the capacity of the health service and watching the actions of decision-makers closely are social attitudes that could be observed not only in the first but also in subsequent phases of the pandemic.

The perception of risks evolved and its axis was the shifting attention – from focusing on one's own health and the health of one's loved ones, to focusing on the organisation of health services, to assessing the state of the economy and government support. It should be stressed that public opinion polls are a kind of photograph of the moods and opinions of the public, influenced by current events. Social surveys related to the assessment of government actions in the first period of the pandemic indicated that the public is divided in its assessment of government decisions. Such a phenomenon can be observed in all V4 countries except Hungary. In Poland, during the first wave, 44% of respondents positively evaluated government decisions, while 46% expressed a negative opinion (CBOS, 55/2020 Assessment of government actions during the pandemic).[3] In the background of the diagnosed polarisation of public opinion was the escalating political dispute over the date of the presidential elections. This also resulted in differentiated evaluations by individual voters, as 93% of those identifying themselves as Law and Justice (Prawo i Sprawiedliwość) vote gave positive ratings of the government's actions, with only 18% of voters of the opposition Civic Coalition (Koalicja Obywatelska).

In the early stages of the pandemic, the focus of the research was to assess the adequacy of government actions to the pandemic situation. It was mentioned earlier that governments may have taken excessive or too restrictive measures or, conversely, underestimated the epidemiological threat through insufficient or no action. In Poland, nearly half of the respondents assessed the introduced restrictions as adequate and appropriate to the situation, while nearly a quarter assessed them as too tough (CBOS, 55/2020). Given the cost of shutting down the economy, a special group were entrepreneurs. During the de facto presidential campaign period, it was in the government's interest to create the impression that it understood what losses entrepreneurs were suffering as a result of the introduced restrictions and was working to offset these losses. Unfortunately, in April 2020, 64% of respondents in Poland expressed fears about the effectiveness of the government's activities in the sphere of the economy, while nearly one-fourth of respondents expressed hope for an improvement in the economic situation as a result of the government's activity (CBOS, 55/2020), with as many as 70% of voters of the United Right (Zjednoczona Prawica) seeing the government's offered assistance as sufficient, and only 3% of the Civic Coalition voters. As many as 90% of government supporters and only 4% of the latter voters saw prospects for economic improvement. We are therefore dealing with the first signs of politicisation of social attitudes towards the actions of the Polish government in the first period of the pandemic.

The first wave of the pandemic was a time of building a space for cooperation between decision-makers and the public, which was characterised by a *clarification of attitudes* both towards the pandemic itself and towards the decisions made by the government. The very subordination to restrictions can be assessed as relatively widespread, which does not change the fact that from the very beginning of the pandemic there were also sceptical attitudes, questioning both the very existence of the virus responsible for it and thus the pandemic itself, as well as the government's actions in this respect. The clarification of attitudes towards government action was fostered by several factors. These included the dissemination of information about what COVID-19 is, the daily statistics provided and the frequent announcements of new legislation. And while the first two factors did not arouse significant controversy, the frequency of communication of changes in the restrictions in the subjective and objective sense, as well as the inconsistency, often fostered divisions in public opinion in the context of assessing the legitimacy and sensibility of the government's decisions. The inconsistency with regard to the rules on wearing masks, closure of certain facilities and even parks and forests resulted in part of the society becoming convinced of the government's incompetence, part considering its actions as excessive, part sharing the government's position on various issues. Surveys conducted by the Public Opinion Research Centre (CBOS) on the evaluation of government activities confirmed the existence of a strong correlation of this evaluation with party sympathies.[4] The decisive factor is therefore the generalised negative attitude towards the ruling parties, and not the mere fact of questioning the sense of restrictions. Thus, further manifestations of the politicisation of social attitudes towards the actions of the government can be observed.

Apart from political sympathies, two other factors correlating with the type of evaluation can be seen – first of all, demographic characteristics. A positive assessment of the government's actions increases with age, lower education level and socio-economic status, as well as with the size of the place of residence – higher in small towns and villages.[5] Fluctuations in the assessment of the government and its actions are also correlated with waves of infections.[6] It can be concluded, therefore, that the social opinion on the effectiveness of the Polish government's activities in fighting the epidemic is more an expression of the attitude towards authority and depends on the party sympathies and general social status of the respondents than the actual effectiveness. In the electorate, the government's efforts are appreciated mainly by supporters of the Law and Justice party (and coalition parties), while most voters of opposition parties have a negative opinion of the effectiveness of the government's actions in the fight against COVID-19. The politicisation of social attitudes towards the government's actions in Poland was therefore reinforced during the pandemic.

In the Czech Republic, the Centre for the Study of Public Opinion (CSVM) in May 2020 reported the results of a survey according to which the government's actions were indicated as adequate by 70% of the respondents, while almost one-fifth considered them too much and only 8% as inadequate. The results of these surveys show that Czechs were more satisfied with the government's actions and more people were convinced of their effectiveness during the first state of emergency (12 March–17 May 2020) than the subsequent ones (CVVM, Naše společnost, září 2020, 5.9.2020–20.9.2020). In May 2020, economic support for various industries of the economy was rated as very good by 60% of Czechs and as too little by 30% (https://cvvm.soc.cas.cz/media/com_form2content/documents/c2/a5380/f9/pi210512.pdf).

The above assessments have changed with the changing dynamic of infections with COVID-19. In the Czech Republic, as in Poland, the assessment of the government's actions is the result of public entanglement in a political dispute. In May 2020, the state of emergency was cancelled, which should be associated, on the one hand, with a flattening of the number of infections and, on the other, with problems in the functioning of the minority government of Prime Minister Andrej Babiš. In addition, the fiscal policy pursued by his cabinet has raised concerns about the political impact of the coming economic recession. Interestingly, another Czech pollster, Kantar, found that the measures introduced by the Babiš government were supported by 80% of Czechs, while the abolition of restrictions was supported by 69%.[7] According to an analysis by the Polish Institute of International Affairs, one of the factors limiting criticism of Babiš's ANO party was the cancellation, due to the ban on all gatherings, of mass anti-government demonstrations that took place across the country last year (Ogrodnik, n.d.).

A sharp drop in positive ratings of the Czech government's actions occurred in February 2021 (to 44%) and remained at a similar level for the following months. The percentage of people rating these actions as insufficient is relatively lower among people with higher education and among those who do not trust the government. Trust in the government is also a factor influencing the assessment of measures to support the economy – those who do not trust the government believe that measures to support the economy are insufficient and the state does little against the spread of the coronavirus. Older people aged 65 are positive about government action, while those aged 25–34 are far less likely to consider measures to support the economy as "adequate".

The Czech public rated the actions of the fire brigade and the army highly – 92% and 87%, respectively, rated them positively, in contrast to the government, whose actions were rated critically by as many as 72%, a significant increase in negative ratings compared to May 2020 – when the figure was 33%. According to Czech respondents, the EU and the Czech crisis staff also performed badly and very badly, with 58% and 55% of the votes, respectively. The Ministry of Health was also not very well evaluated, with only 37% of respondents rating its actions positively against almost 57% of negative evaluations.

Summarising the results of social research carried out in the Czech Republic in the field of mutual perception of threats, restrictions and state aid, one can notice, similarly to Poland, changes in social attitudes. However, the evaluation of support for the economy comes to the fore, mainly due to rising unemployment. Support was assessed as definitely effective or rather effective by 47% in May 2020, 36% in December and 31% in April 2021 (CVVM, Naše společnost, září 2020, 5.9.2020–20.9.2020).

According to Martyna Wasiuta,

> the reason for the changes in the attitude to restrictions and assessment of the government of Andrej Babiš is probably the decline in credibility and trust towards him. These have been brought about by the creation of a false sense of security by the head of the executive as a result of the campaign of the Czech success in the fight against the epidemic after the first wave and the government's inconsistent communication with the public. The Czech Prime Minister in June (2020, EMM's note) assured that the country was prepared for the so-called second wave and at the same time promised that mass restrictions would not be introduced again. What is more, the government's plenipotentiary for healthcare research and later its minister informed on public television that the second wave of the epidemic was unlikely to come.[8] An opinion poll in October showed that only 36 per cent of Czechs trusted Prime Minister Andrej Babiš as a source of information about the epidemic, the least among other institutions (experts and epidemiologists lead, followed by public media).
>
> (Wasiuta, 2020)

The author suggests that

> there has been politicisation of attitudes towards restrictions in the Czech Republic. Some Czechs linked the obligation to obey the restrictions with submission to the authority of a politician they do not support. In other words, voters of opposition parties, as a sign of their dislike for the prime minister against whom they have been protesting for two years, may be less willing to comply with the emergency regulations issued by his government. One example is the wearing of masks. Czechs who declare trust in the government are more likely to see them as an effective prevention tool against coronavirus infection.
>
> (Wasiuta, 2020)

Protests against the restrictions in the Czech Republic have taken place, for example, on 18 October 2020 in Prague, where nearly 2,000 people gathered. The demonstration was called by the newly formed Movement of Civic Discontent (Hnutí občanské nespokojenosti, HON).

In Slovakia, public attention during the first period of the COVID-19 pandemic focused not so much on the pandemic itself as on the state of the economy. Given that Slovakia had coped well with the pandemic at this stage, and in the economic sphere there was a 4.1% drop in GDP in the first quarter of 2020, concern about both the pandemic and the economy was noted in the polls. The polling centre Focus found at the time that Slovaks were similarly concerned about both the pandemic and the effects of a bad economy – 46.3% and 45.4%, respectively. However, a number of measures taken quickly and the introduction of a state of emergency were producing results. Numerous restrictions, including wearing masks, also contributed to controlling the pandemic in its first period. In Slovakia, TV presenters and politicians were wearing masks. The low death rate placed Slovakia at the forefront of European countries coping well with the pandemic.

The Slovak government reacted relatively quickly and decisively to the risk of coronavirus. According to an analyst from the Centre for Eastern Studies (OSW) in Warsaw,

> the general perception is that one of the reasons for this attitude (quick and decisive reaction, author's note) is the poor condition of the Slovak health service, including the shortage and high average age of medical staff (56 years for doctors, more than a third at retirement age), which makes them particularly vulnerable to infection. Shortages of medical equipment are also a problem. The firm steps taken in this situation reflect a lack of confidence in the capacity of the health service in the event of a sudden increase in the number of patients requiring hospital care.
>
> (Dębiec, 2020)

Interestingly, these swift steps were taken by Slovakia's outgoing Prime Minister Peter Pellegrini, whose party was about to move into opposition, bringing into the decision-making process those politicians who would soon form a government coalition. The next cabinet, that of Igor Matovič, could concentrate on fighting the recession. The Slovak prime minister played a major role in the Slavkov Trilateral (the Czech Republic, Slovakia and Austria), which was important in coordinating the border regime and in coordinating sectoral and economic activities during the recovery from recession.[9]

The Slovak public, in a survey by the research agency AKO[10] expressed their opinion on the most acute problems. Thus, "Aid to distressed companies and sole traders" was indicated by 30% of respondents and "Unemployment and labour market" by almost 25% of indications. These areas – according to the respondents – should be considered priorities in the fight against the pandemic. The dominance of topics from the economic area shows that the public is concerned about the state of the Slovak economy and how to combat the economic effects of COVID-19. There is one surprising indication in these surveys – "Corruption" as an issue to be addressed by the government received the recommendation of less than 5% of respondents, although in the past, especially in the pre-election period, this topic was always put in the first place. In the current post-crisis situation, it seems to have lost its importance for citizens.

Slovaks were generally positive about the actions of Health Minister Marek Krajčić. He received good marks among 40% of respondents who said that he fulfils public expectations completely or well, while bad marks only among 25%. Respondents also expressed their opinion on Prime Minister Igor Matovič. Thus, 33.4% of them positively evaluate the fact that he leads the Slovak government, with 38% negative evaluations.[11]

In the case of Slovakia, it can therefore be said that social attitudes, like those in the other analysed countries, are varied when it comes to attitudes towards political leaders, but they are distinguished by their focus on the economic aspects of the functioning of the state.

The subsequent phases of the pandemic showed difficulties of a different kind: with crisis management or the purchase of the Russian vaccine, which eventually led to the fall of the Matovič government and its replacement by the Eduardo Heger government. Matovič was accused of messy communication and chaos in managing the pandemic recovery plan. In February and March 2021, Slovakia struggled with a huge increase in the number of infections and the highest mortality rate, and the number of hospitalisations due to coronavirus was per capita the highest in the world. As one could read in Deusche Welle in February 2021, the Slovak government asked for EU assistance due to the very high number of deaths recorded during this period. In March 2021, among other things, a ban on leaving the house from 8 pm to 1 am and the obligation to wear FFP2 filter masks were introduced. At the same time, the intensity of monitoring of compliance with the restrictions was intensified.[12]

OSW analysts pointed out that the epidemic situation in Slovakia was the result of loosened social discipline and insufficient control of compliance with restrictions. Particular attention was paid to competence chaos, which also translated into inconsistency in government communication with the public and a lack of consultation with epidemiologists. The successes in the fight against the pandemic in the first wave and the speed of the government's response during that period meant that Slovaks encountered the negative effects of COVID-19 only at the beginning of the next wave of the pandemic.[13] The authorities tried to increase the pace of vaccination, appealed for faster and larger supplies of preparations from tranches ordered by the EC and for solidarity from other EU countries. Public opinion was focused on the assessment of the organisation of vaccinations (which is discussed in Section 6.3). An interesting survey on prestige and trust in various institutions can testify to the public mood of Slovaks during this period. It shows that Slovaks trust the Slovak Academy of Sciences the most (74% of respondents) followed by universities (72%), local authorities (70%) and Slovak Radio and Television (63%). Two conclusions can be drawn from these surveys – one of which relates to the appreciation of scientific institutions with enduring prestige developed over many centuries. In situations where certain mechanisms are destabilised, or at least dysfunctional, societies turn to institutions associated with authority. The high ratings for local authorities, as opposed to the government (only 23% positive ratings, the lowest among the institutions surveyed), may indicate that in crisis situations, the authority which is close to the people is better able to manage the crisis, due to its ability to quickly identify problems and difficulties. One can take notice of the high ratings given to the mass media, perhaps perceived as a source of reliable information.[14]

Hungary, like Slovakia, also did well in the first phase of the pandemic. Although a state of emergency was introduced in March 2020, it attracted a lot of comments from international public opinion due to the de facto curtailment of parliamentary functions in favour of governing through decrees. In a period of nearly four months, some 200 decrees and as many regulations were issued, resulting in legal disorder. In addition, some of these decrees were not related to COVID-19 but to economic or political issues.

According to research conducted by the "Nézőpont" Institute, 65% of respondents said they were satisfied with the government's management of the epidemic in the initial period. These surveys also stressed that there was a good chance that the COVID-19 treatment would be a political success for the ruling party (https://nezopont.hu/meg-tobben-elegedettek). Similarly, in the summer of 2020, the same research centre recorded Hungarians' satisfaction with the government's management of the epidemic; 65% of respondents expressed hope for a return to pre-epidemic living conditions, restarting the economy. The availability of vaccines played an important role in the persistence of positive ratings.

> The increase in satisfaction and the cessation of the epidemic is a very positive process for the government. There is a good chance that the management of the epidemic will be a political success for Orbán's fourth government. Satisfaction among supporters of the ruling party rose from 89 to 91% during the week, but there was also an increase in the anti-government camp, with the percentage satisfied with the epidemic treatment rising from 26 to 30% (66% of the dissatisfied).
>
> (Nézőpont, 2021)

In June 2020, the Hungarian government lifted the state of emergency (closure of borders, schools, cinemas and entertainment venues, with restaurants and cafes open only until 3 pm. Later, it also restricted people from going out to the most necessary situations, such as work or shopping) declared in connection with the COVID-19 pandemic and imposed a state of health emergency throughout the country. Some of the steps taken by the government in imposing the state of emergency remained in force (e.g. the operational staff for the fight against COVID-19, the system of uniformed "hospital commanders"). The Coronavirus Protection Act adopted on 30 March, according to which the government could, among other things, suspend the application of certain laws, derogate from the provisions of laws and take other extraordinary steps to guarantee the life and health of citizens and the stability of the national economy, has also lost its validity.

As one could read in Deutsche Welle,

> in reality, the formal lifting of the state of emergency in Hungary is not at all a clear-cut matter. For the parliament in Budapest has announced the end of the extraordinary powers enjoyed by the prime minister during the state of emergency, but at the same time it has passed a new law on the so-called state of medical emergency. This neologism means in practice the introduction of a new state of emergency in Hungary, during which Victor Orbán will continue to be able to rule by decrees, which will be even more difficult for anyone to control than before.
>
> (Verseck, 2020)

The imposition of a state of medical emergency triggered a number of critical comments, particularly from NGOs, the Hungarian Helsinki Committee, or the Hungarian Union for Human Rights (TASZ), and the Hungarian branch of Amnesty International, which unanimously stated that the government would continue to be able to rule by decree without minimum constitutional safeguards. Restrictions on journalists' access to information and data protection were maintained. Local authorities were deprived of tax revenues and other sources of their income were reduced. This applies particularly to towns and municipalities governed by representatives of the opposition. The action against them is also aimed at limiting the financing of political parties' activities, since tax-funded political campaigns are mainly conducted in Hungary by Prime Minister Orbán's government, not his Fidesz party (Verseck, 2020).

In the subsequent phases of the pandemic, the focus of the relationship between policymakers and the public shifted to the issues of vaccination and economic assessment. The entanglement of the fight against COVID-19 with the escalating political dispute, the dominance of statements discrediting political opponents in the governmental media and especially on the Hungarian left, and on the other hand, the popularisation of the view that it was only thanks to Orbán's efficiency that Hungary was winning the fight against the pandemic – also contributed to the politicisation of the pandemic, which was visible more on the party scene than in public opinion. Good economic indicators in Hungary are directing public attention to ways of dealing with the post-pandemic economic crisis – rather than to health issues, which Hungary has handled relatively well.

From the research presented, certain social attitudes emerge as a result of government actions. In the first period of COVID-19 they were characterised by submissiveness to the actions of the authorities and acceptance of decisions related mainly to restrictions. Gradually, however, in view of the identified sequential and simultaneous incoherence – doubts emerged in these societies as to the rightness and sensibility of individual decisions. Chaos crept into the decision-making process, marked not only by inconsistencies in the management of the pandemic crisis but also by the political situation and tensions arising within it. In Poland, the dynamics of the situation were created by the timing of presidential elections, in Slovakia by the change in the prime minister's seat, and in the Czech Republic by the problems associated with the minority government. Attitudes to the decisions of those in power began to take on a political character, i.e. acceptance vs. negation of these decisions was mediated by a generalised positive or negative attitude to authority. A degree of ambivalence and even confusion emerged in attitudes. This manifested itself in both the understanding of threats and social behaviour.

## 6.3 Identification of public attitudes towards vaccination

A new phase in the government's cooperation with society took place during the introduction and continuation of vaccinations. Social attitudes towards vaccination are the result of several factors. The cognitive component of attitudes prompts us to look for their origins in knowledge about vaccination and vaccines as disease prevention agents. In this case there is a competition between scientific knowledge (medical knowledge) and common knowledge (common sense), often the result of established opinions and beliefs. Secondly, attitudes may derive from the observation of other societies that have already largely been vaccinated and the resulting benefits. Thirdly, attitudes to vaccination are shaped by emotions. The COVID-19 vaccine aroused particular emotions, including fear and apprehension of adverse post-vaccination reactions, but on the other hand, it also aroused positive emotions, and above all hope that the possibility of a return to normality, often referred to as the "new normal", would be created. It is therefore worth focusing not so much on the sources of the attitudes themselves but on the question of what these attitudes are. In March 2021, several months after the first vaccinations, the attitudes of the populations in the V4 countries towards vaccination were examined.

In the first decade of March 2021, the Slovak research agency Focus surveyed the populations of the Visegrad countries on behalf of the Budapest-based think tank Political Capital, and identified attitudes towards vaccination. "Anybody who raised concerns about the jabs was immediately labelled as an 'anti-vaxxer' or 'conspiracy theorist', while those who do reject vaccination refused to listen to any rational argument that may challenge their convictions", the authors write in the introduction to the study. They thus suggest that these attitudes are not two-dimensional – for or against – but more complex. This reflection should discourage the simple classification of people into pro- or anti-vaccination groups. As a result of this research, five attitudes towards vaccination have been identified that reflect this complexity:

- *Anti-vaxxers*: people who would not be vaccinated against the coronavirus because they agree with the statement that vaccines cause more problems than they solve;[15]

- *General vaccine sceptics*: people who agree with the statement on vaccines but would choose to vaccinate or have already done so;
- *COVID-19 vaccine sceptics*: respondents who are generally not against vaccination but still would not vaccinate against COVID-19;
- *Vaccine supporters*: respondents who disagree with the above statement regarding vaccinations and are certain that they would take COVID-19 or have already done so;
- *Uncertain respondents*: this relatively heterogeneous group does not fit a definite category on vaccines in general and is divided in their views on taking the COVID-19 vaccine (Political Capital, 2021).

The results of these surveys allow the construction of country-specific vaccine profiles. The discrepancy between countries in terms of definite "anti-vaxxers" in the population is relatively large: 14% of Poles, only 4% of Hungarians and 8.6% of Slovaks and 10.3% of Czechs belong here (Political Capital, 2021).

The distribution of attitudes towards the COVID-19 vaccine is somewhat different. Among the opponents of vaccination against COVID-19 there are 11.6% of Slovaks, 15.7% of Poles, 17.8% of Czechs and 17.9% of Hungarians. Thus, the generalised dislike of vaccination – low among Hungarians – only 4%, does not translate into an attitude to one against COVID-19 – more than four times as many "anti-COVID-vaxxers". The percentage of "supporters of vaccination" and acceptance of any vaccine is by far the lowest in the Czech Republic (only 18%), in Poland almost twice as high (36.5%). In Slovakia the propensity to vaccinate is the highest at 51.6%, similarly in Hungary – 50.5% (Political Capital, 2021). These data reveal certain characteristics of the nations discussed. The Czechs are the most hesitant about vaccinations, the Slovaks and the Hungarians are the most supportive of vaccinations in general, and the level of scepticism about vaccination against COVID-19 is similar in three countries – Poland, the Czech Republic and Hungary – while the highest number of anti-vaxxers is in Poland and the Czech Republic.

The Slovak Focus also investigated, on behalf of Political Capital, the general propensity to vaccinate in the analysed countries. It found that it is associated with trust in one's government or health authority.

> Our regional research also showed that this is not a national characteristic. In all countries studied, the average propensity to vaccinate is higher among people who trust official institutions more than those who do not. This is particularly pronounced in Hungary and Poland. The most willing to vaccinate are those who trust the authorities and those who do not trust them do not want to vaccinate.
>
> (Political Capital, 2021)

Regardless of the country studied, respondents had a similar view on vaccination, but in the Czech Republic the opinion is not so clear-cut, while

Slovaks are characterised by exceptional trust in the Russian vaccine. The percentage of those who refuse vaccination (who definitely do not want to or rather will not be vaccinated) ranges from 20 to 29 in the Visegrad countries. Poles and Czechs have the highest anti-vaccination rates: 29% and 28%, respectively, definitely or rather reject vaccination. Among Hungarians and Slovaks the percentage of those reluctant to vaccinate is 22% and 20%, respectively (Political Capital, 2021).

In Poland in April 2021, 65% of adult Poles declared a positive attitude to vaccination against COVID-19, compared to 36% in November and 57% in January 2021 (CBOS, Attitude to vaccination against COVID-19 and evaluation of their organisation, 50/2021). The authors of the study write that

> the analysis of socio-demographic differences shows that a more favourable attitude to vaccination is declared by residents of the largest cities (only 13% do not want to be vaccinated), university graduates (22% do not want to be vaccinated) and respondents from households with the highest per capita income – at least PLN 3,000 (16% do not want to be vaccinated).
>
> (CBOS, 50/2021)

The profile of the person declaring vaccination described in this way coincides with the demographic characteristics of the supporters of the opposition and not of the ruling coalition in Poland. The analysis of the vaccination map in Poland and the map depicting the electoral preferences indicates a certain paradox, however, under the assumption that the level of vaccination in individual regions in Poland is the result of the appeals of those in power and their COVID-19 control policy and not of an individual decision based on a high level of health awareness. It can therefore be concluded that the efforts of those in power are not being responded to by people who are their voters, report high levels of trust in "their" parties in other surveys and yet do not make the decision to vaccinate.

One can therefore conclude that the relationship (examined by Political Capital) between the propensity to vaccinate and trust in the government is not fully confirmed in the case of Poland. Naturally – and this should be stressed once again – individual motivations and inclination to rational action, rather than political sympathies, may play an important role here. While we are dealing with a politicisation of attitudes towards government decisions in general, as they are filtered by party preferences, this phenomenon can no longer be diagnosed in attitudes towards vaccination in Poland. In late April 2021, the Hungarian portal nezopont.hu published a study by the "Nézőpont" Institute showing that 64% of Hungarians said they were satisfied with the government's vaccination plan. Even 37% of the government's critics said so. Seventy-three per cent of those surveyed no longer report the fear of eastern vaccines and agree that any vaccine is better than a disease, while 22% disagree with such a statement (Nézőpont, 2021).

The pro-government portal Szazadveg.hu, presenting a study from March 2021, even goes into raptures over the Orbán government's policy in connection with the organisation of vaccinations. The success of vaccinations is connected to the fact that five vaccines are allowed in Hungary and to the policy of vaccinating as many people as possible with the first dose, as well as the creation of vaccination centres in many towns (Węgry, 2021). As you can read on this website "these outstanding results were achieved by health workers during the third wave, when the number of cases reached its peak". Fifty-eight per cent of Hungarians expressed satisfaction with the vaccination process in this survey The Szazadveg survey further shows that Hungarians are critical of the EU's policy towards the purchase of vaccines – 52% criticise this policy, with 37% believing that the EU is not responsible for the purchase of vaccines.

The attitudes of V4 societies towards vaccination are therefore diverse, subject to dynamics over time. The interest and declarations during the initial period of vaccine availability did not coincide with the actual state of the number of people vaccinated in each country.

## 6.4 Mediatisation of the pandemic – psychological, cultural and political challenges

Mediatisation is the process of including the media in various spheres of social life and a specific modification of these spheres through the media. On the one hand, specific social objectives are achieved through the media, while the media provide a forum for public discourse, initiating a debate on socially important issues and, in accordance with the normative function, and promote certain socially desirable patterns of behaviour. The pandemic situation poses serious challenges to the media in this respect.

The assumption that the media have an overwhelming influence on shaping the attitudes and views of their recipients has been present in the literature on this subject for many years (Mrozowski, 2001, pp. 357–392). Putting these issues in a necessary nutshell, it should be noted that the media, by setting the agenda, indicate what elements, facts and events the recipients should pay attention to and suggest what is important and worth interpreting on a given day. They also suggest how to interpret these facts, situating them in a specific interpretative framework. This means that the media cannot be viewed through the prism of their primary function, which is to disseminate information. Media should also be seen as an active entity that shapes the opinions of their audience.

The claim that in crisis situations the role of the media increases refers not only to traditional media (radio, television, press) but also to social media. During crises, the media not only inform but also shape people's views, opinions and behaviour to a much greater extent than in normal times. Although it is the informational and creative function of the media that dominates in times of crisis, other classic functions – educational or mobilising – should not be forgotten either. A special role in this respect should be attributed to social media. Toni G.L.A van der Meer and Piet Verhoeven (2013) in their article "Public framing organisational crisis situations: Social media versus news media" point out that public social media, especially "tweets", play an important role in shaping the course of a crisis. Through them the course of the crisis can be shaped, escalated, or prevented. A similar role can be attributed to Facebook, which has been used by public figures responsible for decision-making and dissemination of information on various topics related to the corona crisis.

In times of crisis, social media provide an opportunity for effective communication, especially for politicians or opinion leaders. Unfortunately, the activity of social media during the coronavirus pandemic also revealed its negative sides, which are worth mentioning. There was, for example, a lot of false information, and in some countries there were even attempts to monopolise the communication of decision-makers with the public and even to penalise independent activity in the media.

With regard to the period in question, one can point to the increased activity of the media in the countries under study, which became widely involved in the process of disseminating information and shaping attitudes towards COVID-19. In the first days of March alone, there were 1.1 million mentions of COVID-19 in the Polish media and 235,000 mentions in the traditional media.[16] The fact that members of the public were looking for and using information published in the media is evidenced by the significant increase in the number of visits on various portals. For example, the top ten Polish news portals recorded a 57% increase in the number of visitors[17]

Unfortunately, these increases in online media consumption have not always translated into an increase in the quality of public information on the pandemic, which is in line with the general trends outlined in the introduction. In fact, one could argue that there has been a disproportionate increase in fake news. The Press Service counted that during the first phase of the pandemic, numerous fake news stories were disseminated concerning, for example, the treatment of coronavirus. The most common of these referred to the effectiveness of administering vitamin C, drinking water every 15 minutes, or drinking alcohol.[18] Some online newspapers in Central and Eastern Europe (CEE) saw their number of visitors increase by 1,000%, reaching their highest ever number of users and page views.

The initial period of the pandemic brought disturbing phenomena related to the restriction of access to data on the pandemic by governments, which, while protecting their monopoly in this area, also restricted citizens' freedom of access to information. For example, doctors in Poland and Hungary reported that they were banned from talking to media representatives about coronavirus under threat of dismissal or fines, especially when they pointed out shortages in protective equipment for health workers. In Poland, professor Simon was banned from speaking to the media in this way. In Hungary, several university professors admitted that they were banned from speaking to the media, and journalists who criticised the government's handling of the pandemic received death threats via emails or through social media.[19] In response, many independent online services opened up free access to their articles on coronavirus and public health measures so that there was no inequality in access to reliable information. Thanks to online access, everyone could access them without much trouble (Zbytniewska, 2021).

In Poland, many media institutions have changed their broadcasting schedules and special information and advice programmes have been introduced.[20] In Hungary some Internet portals have become guide services. There, one could find information on how to deal with various special situations both professional and private related to COVID-19. For example, the portal https://tasz.hu/koronavirus was set up in 1994 and basically promotes human rights and disseminates information on how to defend oneself against unjustified interventions and omissions of the authorities.[21] In the Czech Republic, mojemedicina.cz, an internet portal accessible to anyone interested in health and medicine, has a lot of content related to COVID-19 as does the popular portal seznam.cz. In Slovakia, there is a portal adanity. sk, which publishes various content related to COVID-19.

The presented examples clearly show that media – in line with the aforementioned paradigm of the active role of the media – provide the public not only with topics but also with ways of interpreting them. It is also possible to observe the activity of media audiences themselves, with regard to obtaining information about COVID-19, which is well illustrated by Czech research. Almost two-thirds (65%) of Czechs monitored information about the coronavirus in traditional media at least once a day in April, 41% once a day, 16% followed media events once every few days, 5% once a week, 6% less than once a week, and 8% of Czech citizens did not follow them at all. Websites, blogs, discussion forums or social networks were visited several times a day by 20% of the population, once a day by 28%, by 14% once every few days, and 22% did not follow online events at all. Coronavirus-related issues were also a frequent topic of everyday conversations. Thus, 16% of respondents talked about it several times a day, and 22%, once a day.

In Poland, interest in COVID-19 is evidenced by record-breaking results of viewing portals dealing with health, including zdrowie.pap.pl portal. The peak of Poles' interest in the new coronavirus came at the turn of February and March 2020. At that time, the Zdrowie portal had up to 50,000 page views a day, and from the beginning of the year to June 2020, the zdrowie. pap.pl portal had a record-breaking 3.3 million page views. Google Analytics data shows, however, that, starting from May, the hunger for information on the new coronavirus started to decrease rapidly in Poland.[22]

The large amount of information that flooded the media led to a certain information chaos. Some of the media recipients developed a gap in knowledge, a certain deficit in information, which required supplementation. In this reduction of cognitive deficits, an invaluable role was played by doctors – medical experts who, despite certain difficulties (already indicated in this article), took on the responsibility to educate the societies about coronavirus. Daily appearances in mass media and significant activity in social media caused medical experts to gradually become new actors of public communication, not only complementary to political leaders but even more trusted compared to politicians. In the Czech Republic, epidemiologists such as Petr Smejkal and Rastislav Maďar, but also biochemist Jan Konvalinka and virologist Ruth Tachezy, became popular medical authorities. In Poland, social research conducted in early 2021 indicated the growing authority of doctors of various specialities educating on COVID-19 issues in the mass media. The IBRIS survey report shows that doctors are more trusted than ministers responsible for the fight against COVID-19. Thus, in January 2021, the trust in doctors active in the media was at the level of 60–65%, (doctor Paweł Grzesiowski – immunologist, Professor Włodzimierz Gut – virologist, Professor Krzysztof Simon – infectious diseases doctor) while the confidence in ministers active in the media was lesser than 30% (IBRIS, study conducted on 18.01.2021 for the newspaper *Fakt*). This result may be interpreted as a premise leading to the conclusion that the process of communication between the government and the public needs to be strengthened by medical experts who are positively evaluated, despite still not being well recognisable at the moment. Their daily activity both in traditional and social media contributes to the widening of the audience, which may be a sign of positive thinking on the change of attitudes towards COVID-19 in the field of prevention and vaccination. A significant distractor in the formation of pro-health attitudes is the heterogeneity of views on some issues – for example, the effectiveness of amantadine treatment. On the other hand, there is hope for a unified and coherent position on vaccination.

An interesting phenomenon in the process of communicating pandemic-related decisions is the emergence of a specific narrative. On the one hand, the information process had a *technocratic* character. Here, the data, numbers, appeals to the factual content of the messages and science-based evidence predominated. An example of such a narrative can be press conferences, where pure information comes to the fore. The main actors of public communication are spokespersons of various institutions, as well as medical experts providing factual knowledge about COVID-19. The second narrative trend is the excessive *axiologisation of communication* by referring to community and national values, which is most evident in Poland and Hungary. Victor Orbán's statements refer to the nation, the value of the family, and the subordination of decisions for the sake of Hungarian families. In Mateusz Morawiecki's statements, such are also visible: "let us protect ourselves and our families, life is an inalienable value". Another feature of the communication of political leaders was the excessive use of emphasis, solemnity – i.e. a kind of statement *pomposity*. Such communication techniques (axiologisation and pomposity) have a high persuasive value and are typical of political leaders. They are designed to activate support for the government in connection with the management of the COVID-19 crisis. In conclusion, it can be said that the media fulfilled its role, not only as a carrier of information but also as a creator of different interpretations of facts and events and an arena for the exchange of views.

After more than a year's experience of fighting COVID-19, various challenges of a psychological but also more broadly cultural and political nature emerge. This relatively short time has been full of experiences, including those of a borderline nature (illness and death of loved ones). The time after the pandemic is and will be the time of regaining *social trust* first and foremost, and repeatedly of building trust anew. With reference to Piotr Sztompka's concept of social trust, it may be indicated that trust is built on the foundations of credibility, cooperation and trust, and its addressees are other people as well as institutions (Sztompka, 2007). The relational character of trust should also be emphasised. And it is from a relational perspective that psychological, cultural and political challenges can be identified at several levels: micro, meso and macro levels. The micro level refers to the closest relationships, family and colleagues, which have been suspended by the lack of possibility of face-to-face contact. It is at this level that the challenge is to regain the feeling of safety resulting from close contact. It is also at this level (for part of the population) that the lost proactivity has to be nurtured. After a period of a kind of helplessness resulting from the need to conform, learning to influence effectively, achieving new goals seems to be the beginning of a new activity.

The meso level is about rebuilding relations with the wider environment, for example, professional or institutional. It is about trust as a cultural rule. The macro level is about building trust in political authority and state institutions. The new normality is at the same time a different normality. It requires strengthening social competences for cooperation and compromise. It is also about institutional initiatives of governments supporting the psychological and cultural condition of people after the experience of corona-crisis and unwanted isolation.

Raised in a climate of distrust of politicians, scepticism about democratic institutions and disillusionment with how democratic processes work, citizens are less and less interested in politics and become less and more superficially engaged in politics. The growing lack of trust in politicians and political institutions results in citizens turning away from formal politics, which in the long run is extremely harmful for democracy, especially in crisis situations, such as the ones being faced since the beginning of 2020. The lack of opportunities for citizens to become politically active has exacerbated the lack of trust in politicians, and this not only undermines faith in existing political solutions but also destroys community patterns of thinking. Unfortunately, the media during the pandemic indirectly contributed to this by maintaining a negative image of the government and the process of governing in the media content – as they are more willing to show its failures and operational ineffectiveness. This simplistic and deformed image of politics is a consequence of the pursuit of viewers who can be attracted by sensationalism and entertainment. It is difficult to give a clear answer to the question: whether and to what extent the media have failed in communicating the essence of politics as an art of negotiation and making difficult choices in the face of crisis. Surely, however, with such an entrenched simplified image of politics and naively understood individualism, citizens are beginning to lack the competences necessary for a collective approach to problems and decision-making. "People distance themselves from politics and become frustrated in their actions because they do not understand the fundamental nature of politics" (Stoker, 2006, p. 184). In the public sphere, it is not enough to be informed and take part in voting – it also takes the ability to listen. Communication, not just casting a vote, is the pinnacle of political competence. The vote is the key currency in democratic politics, but before we cast it, we have to consider who or what solution to vote for, and then the ability to listen is crucial. Politics is the art of taking account of different points of view and coming to common judgements. Politics is not just a simple manifestation of one's own interest but an attempt to reconcile it with the interests of others, i.e. to overcome social and economic barriers. Resistance is part of politics and creates space for compromise.

Politics in general and democratic politics in particular cannot be based on mobilising people around single issues because such activity is more viral and anarchic in nature. The pandemic should make it clear that politics has become more transnational than it has ever been, while our political institutions and patterns of governance have remained stubbornly national in essence. Besides, in order to cope with the inherently multi-level nature of the modern world and the associated demands of its governance, politics cannot be presented as a pathogen for which de-politicisation is the antidote. Unfortunately, this is not accompanied by an awareness of the socially dangerous consequences of disseminating such a vision of politics – it leads to the destruction of the public sphere. The globalised world, in which we live, is a product of the often unintended interactions between strategies pursued by actors at different levels of multi-level politics. It is extremely difficult to identify key decision-makers and to reconstruct the process of political decision-making, let alone to control them democratically. In politics, globalisation has become almost synonymous with capitulation explaining the need to de-politicise and delegate decision-making powers to independent, external and expert actors largely outside effective public control. Meanwhile, modern political governance is about steering in the context of complexity and unpredictability – the emergence of new political stakeholders and challenges. Unfortunately, our traditional models of democratic thinking do not fit into this reality (Hay & Stoker, 2009, pp. 229–233).

Revitalisation of politics understood more broadly than technocratic governance would require a return to collective forms of decision-making. Citizens need to regain a sense of real influence on the process of making decisions that affect them, which would contribute to rebuilding an understanding of politics as a sphere of social choices. This would help to restore their sense of involvement in public life and to understand some of the measures taken by governments to combat the effects caused by the emergence of the SARS-CoV-2 virus. Unfortunately, the pandemic seems to have perpetuated rather than helped to overcome the culture of anti-politics. The anti-vaccine movement is an expression of resistance to the dominance of one narrative. It is an attempt to politicise a public space that has been appropriated by non-democratically elected professionals and experts. In such a defined space, any anti-government activity can be presented as socially harmful, as it prevents the adoption of solutions presented as effective, in technocratic terms, for a given problem. Unfortunately, the activity of governments and the media during the pandemic confirms that communicative rationality, although needed in politics and even necessary in new and crisis situations, is definitely in retreat in the 21st-century world. Neither politicians nor citizens can change this, even with the use of increasingly modern means of communication, because this requires the spread of a culture of trust and cooperation.

## Notes

1 The decision to close or open schools depending on the age of the pupils, or sports facilities depending on who uses them (professional or amateur athletes), are examples of inconsistency over time due to the surprising timing of implemented changes.
2 In addition, some orders, such as the number of passengers on public transport, were impossible to comply with.
3 The background to this polarisation of public opinion was the escalating political dispute over the timing of the presidential elections. This also affected the differing opinions of individual electorates. Ninety-three per cent of those identifying themselves as Law and Justice voters assessed the government's actions positively, with only 18% of positive assessment by voters of the Civic Coalition. Nearly half of the respondents evaluated the introduced restrictions as adequate and appropriate for the situation, while almost a quarter assessed them as excessive. (CBOS, 55/2020).
4 Supporters of the opposition parties were negatively inclined towards the introduced restrictions, while voters of the ruling United Right overwhelmingly found them adequate.
5 People in the 65+ age cohort are 71% positive about the government's actions, compared to 33% of those aged 18–24. More often than average, people with elementary education (75%) and basic vocational education (69%), respondents in moderate and poor circumstances – with monthly per capita income below PLN 2,000 (62%), as well as residents of rural areas (59%, including farmers – 66%) and small towns (61%) are satisfied with the policies of the government in office. Respondents with higher education (50%), people who are relatively well-off – with a monthly per capita income of at least PLN 3,000 (57%) – and inhabitants of big cities (52%) are most likely to disapprove of government measures (CBOS, Obawy przed zarażeniem się koronawirusem i ocena działań rządu w maju, 60/2021).
6 In May 2021 the government's actions were assessed as definitely good or good by 53% (this is a time of decreasing infections), which is a significant increase compared to March 2021 when the approval of the government's actions was 45% with 50% of negative assessments.
7 According to a Kantar poll from May 2020, Babiš's party could count on 34% support (it received 29.6% of the vote in the 2017 parliamentary elections).

8  Also contributing to undermining the government's credibility was a ruling by the Prague Municipal Court on 23 April 2020. It questioned the legitimacy of four orders restricting retail and service trade (closure of shops, cosmetic establishments, etc.) and freedom of movement during the first state of emergency. They were issued by the Minister of Health and therefore not in accordance with the provisions of the Crisis Management Act, which confers these powers on the government and not on individual members of the government. Key restrictions were therefore invalidated for formal reasons, which could have undermined the image of the government with insufficient understanding of the law in the face of the epidemic.

9  Ogrodnik Ł. *Słowacja w walce z pandemią COVID-19 i jej skutkami dla gospodarki.* Polski Instytut Spraw Międzynarodowych. 9.07.2020.

10  AKO. *Čo ľudia odkazujú vláde? Akým oblastiam sa má vláda prioritne venovať po koronakríze? Výsledky reprezentatívneho prieskumu verejnej mienky.* AKO. sk.

11  *Exkluzívny prieskum: Matovič nezvláda riadenie. Sulíkovo riešenie covidu je najdôveryhodnejšie.* Trend.sk, 1.12.2020.

12  Pędziwol A.M. *Covid-19: Słowacja prosi o pomoc,* Deutsche Welle, 17.02.2021.

13  By the end of August 2020, Slovakia had cumulatively – per capita – 7 times fewer deaths due to COVID-19 than the Czech Republic and more than 50 times fewer than the EU average, had not acquired collective immunity to COVID-19. This created good conditions for the spread of the more infectious so-called UK mutation of the pathogen.

14  Armed Forces of the Slovak Republic (63%) and the president who is trusted by 56%, trade unions (55%), government agencies (51%), police (48%), NGOs (42%) and commercial media (39%) are at the centre of the trust ranking. According to respondents, the least trustworthy is the government, trusted by 23% of respondents. Also at the bottom of the trustworthiness ranking are the National Council (27%), the courts and legal system (31%) and large companies and corporations, which are trusted by 38% of respondents. *Najdôveryhodnejšou inštitúciou na Slovensku je Slovenská akadémia vied. Najmenšiu dôveryhodnosť má vláda,* SME.sk, 16.04.2021.

15  Respondents were asked to respond to this statement by rating a 5-point "agree–disagree" scale.

16  *Koronawirus – raport medialny. 1.01.2020–10.03.2020.*

17  *Skok odwiedzalności serwisów informacyjnych: Onet przed WP, RMF24.pl przed Wyborcza.pl i RadioZET.pl (TOP10)* (2020). wirtualnemedia.pl, 19.03.

18  *Koronawirus – raport medialny. 1.01.2020–10.03.2020.*

19  Hungary's pro-government parliamentary majority further restricted freedom of expression by tightening the criminal code concerning the early stages of the state of emergency. In addition, the freedom to report independently on the epidemic was restricted because reporting on the problems could be seen as "fear-mongering", punishable by up to five years in prison. However, "nobody knew what kind of opinion could be considered a crime", explains Gábor Polyák, associate professor at the University of Pécs. After the law came into force, there were "coordinated attacks and threats against independent media accused of misinformation, although they reported on COVID-19 more responsibly than the pro-government media", according to Reporters Without Borders. Poland has not introduced similar legislation, but two journalists from media critical of the government were accused of violating social distancing rules while covering a protest in front of the Law and Justice leader's home in early May 2020 (https://www.euractiv.pl/section/demokracja/linksdossier/pandemia-koronawirus-media-europa-polska-czechy-wegry-slowacja-bialorus-rosja-ukraina/).

20 Among others, TVN24 started broadcasting the programme "Help yourself – your job" ("Pomagajmy sobie – twoja praca"), featuring the labour market during the epidemic. The host, together with experts, discussed government aid packages which were supposed to limit the economic effects of the epidemic, especially on the labour market. Krajowa Rada Radiofonii i Telewizji (2020). *Zmiany ramówek, audycje specjalne, zawieszone produkcje, łączenia online*. 15.04.2020.
21 On the pages of this portal there is also an evaluation of the vaccination policy, which states that Orban's organisation of vaccinations is not conducive to achieving a reasonable level of vaccination in small towns and villages and among those living in deep poverty.
22 Szczepaniak (2020) W. *Koronawirus w mediach: COVID COVIDA COVIDEM pogania*. Serwis Zdrowie. 10.06.2020.

## References

Boin, A., Lodge, M., & Luesink, M. (2020). Learning the Covid-19 crisis: an initial of national responses. *Policy Design and Practice*, 3, pp. 189–204,

Dębiec, K. (2020). *Słowacja wobec pandemii koronawirusa: płynna zmiana gabinetu*, Ośrodek Studiów Wschodnich, 18.03. Available from: https://www.osw. waw.pl/pl/publikacje/analizy/2020-03-18/slowacja-wobec-pandemii-koronawirusa-plynna-zmiana-gabinetu

Hay, C. (2007). *Why We Hate Politics*. Cambridge: Polity Press.

Hay, C., & Stoker, G. (2009). Revitalising politics: Have we lost the plot. *Representation*, 45(3), pp. 225–236. https://doi.org/10.1080/00344890903129681

Jenkins, L. (2011). The difference genealogy makes: strategies for politicization or how to extend capacities for autonomy. *Political Studies*, 59(1), pp. 156–174. https://doi.org/10.1111/j.1467-9248.2010.00844.x

Karwat, M. (2012). *O karykaturze polityki*. Warszawskie Wydawnictwo Literackie Muza SA.

Krajowa Rada Radiofonii I Telewizji (2020). *Zmiany ramówek, audycje specjalne, zawieszone produkcje, łączenia online*. 15.04. https://www.gov.pl/web/krrit/zmiany-ramowek-audycje-specjalne-zawieszone-produkcje-laczenia-online

Krastew, I., & Holmes, S. (2020). *Światło, które zgasło. Jak Zachód zawiódł swoich wyznawców*. Warszawa: Wydawnictwo Krytyki Politycznej.

Maj, K., & Skarżyńska, K. (2020). *Społeczeństwo wobec epidemii. Raport z adan.* Available from: https://www.batory.org.pl/wp-content/uploads/2020/04/Badanie-spoleczenstwo-wobec-epidemii _fin.pdf

Mrozowski, M. (2001). *Media masowe. Władza, rozrywka, biznes*. Warszawa: Oficyna Wydawnicza Aspra.

Ogrodnik, Ł. (n.d.). *Czeska awangarda – sposoby radzenia sobie z epidemią COVID-19*, PISM Biuletyn nr 108.

*Skok odwiedzalności serwisów informacyjnych: Onet przed WP, RMF24.pl przed Wyborcza.pl I RadioZET.pl (TOP10)* (2020). Wirtualnemedia.pl, 19.03. Avalilable from: https://www.wirtualnemedia.pl/artykul/koronawirus-epidemia-skok-odwiedzalnosci-serwisow-informacyjnych-onet-przed-wp-rmf24-pl-przed-wyborcza-pl-i-radiozet-pl-top10

Stoker, G. (2006). Politics in mass democracies: destined to disappoint? *Representation*, 42(3), pp. 181–194.

Szczepaniak W. (2020). *Koronawirus w mediach: COVID COVIDA COVIDEM pogania*. Serwis Zdrowie. 10.06. Available from: https://zdrowie.pap.pl/blog/byc-zdrowym/koronawirus-w-mediach-covid-covida-covidem-pogania

Sztompka, P. (2007). *Zaufanie. Fundament społeczeństwa*. Kraków: Wydawnictwo Znak.

Wasiuta, M. (2020). *Czeska opinia publiczna wobec działań rządu w ramach walki z epidemią Covid-19*, Przemiany Ustrojowe, 4.11. Available from: http://przemianyustrojowe.pl/eseje/czeska-opinia-publiczna-wobec-dziaa-rzdu-w-ramach-walki-z-epidemi-covid-19

Van der Meer, Toni GLA, & Verhoeven, Piet (2013). Public framing Organisational crisis situations: Social media versus news media. *Public Relations Review*, 39(3), pp. 229–231.

Verseck, K. (2020). *Węgry: Zniesienie stanu wyjątkowego niewiele zmieni*. Deutsche Welle. 17.06. Available from: https://www.dw.com/pl/w%C4%99gry-zniesienie-stanu-wyj%C4%85tkowego-niewiele-zmieni/a-53842855

Węgry (2021). Węgry zostały mistrzem Europy w szczepieniach. *Die Welt*, March 2021. Available from: Zbytniewska K. (2021). *Koronawirus a media: Jak pandemia COVID-19 wpłynęła na wolność słowa i sytuację mediów w Europie Srodkowo-Wschodniej?* EURACTIV.pl. 13.03. Available from: https://www.euractiv.pl/section/demokracja/linksdossier/pandemia-koronawirus-media-europa-polska-czechy-wegry-slowacja-bialorus-rosja-ukraina/

### Social surveys

AKO https://ako.sk/wp-content/uploads/2020/06/Co_ludia_odkazuju_vlade.pdf

AKO https://ako.sk/wp-content/uploads/2020/12/ag.AKO-Prieskum-verejnej-mienky.pdf.

CBOS https://www.cbos.pl/SPISKOM.POL/2020/K_055_20.PDF

CBOS https://www.cbos.pl/SPISKOM.POL/2021/K_050_21.PDF

CBOS https://www.cbos.pl/SPISKOM.POL/2021/K_060_21.PDF

CSVM, *Naše společnost – září 2020* (5.09. – 20.09.) https://cvvm.soc.cas.cz/cz/tiskove-zpravy/politicke/instituce-a-politici/5299-hodnoceni-reakce-a-pripravenosti-statu-a-jeho-instituci-na-epidemii-covid-19-nase-spolecnost-zari-2020.

CSVM, *Naše společnost – speciál – duben 2021* https://cvvm.soc.cas.cz/cz/tiskove-zpravy/politicke/instituce-a-politici/5379-hodnoceni-reakce-instituci-na-epidemii-covid-19-a-dodrzovani-opatreni-proti-sireni-koronaviru-nase-spolecnost-special-duben-2021

CSVM, *Naše společnost – speciál – duben 2021* https://cvvm.soc.cas.cz/media/com_form2content/documents/c2/a5380/f9/pi210512.pdf

Nezopont https://nezopont.hu/csucsot-dontott-az-oltaspartisag/

SzazadveG https://szazadveg.hu/en/2021/06/08/downturn-on-an-annual-basis-growth-on-a-quarterly-basis~n1883

Political Capital https://www.politicalcapital.hu/hirek.php?article_read=1&article_id=2759

# 7 The situation and role of the armed forces during the pandemic

*Jacek Dworzecki, Mojmír Mamojka, and Lucia Kurilovská*

The role of the armed forces is to have a military potential allowing, in case of such necessity, to effectively protect the territory of one's own country and to respond to all kinds of threats, not only of military but also of asymmetric character. It should be noted that the areas of activity of contemporary armed forces – including on the plane of civil operations – are definitely more numerous. Therefore, the armed forces are subject to constant transformations in the area of organisation, technology or development of human resources.

The influence of the armed forces on the realities of socio-political life is visible in many internal aspects of the functioning of every democratic state. Today it is difficult to imagine the conduct of activities by the civilian state administration in responding to serious crisis situations without the participation of the military component. Of course, the state has at its disposal the police or rescue services, but in many situations, the capabilities of these services (especially the technical ones) are not sufficient to remove threats of non-military nature that have arisen.

The armed forces in a modern state possess certain specific features which allow, among other things, to undertake even the most complex actions in response to the occurrence of events defined as crisis situations. The most important feature describing the specificity of the armed forces, which is not present in other civilian organisations, is operational autonomy. The armed forces can take immediate action at any time regardless of the circumstances. This is possible thanks to many components and solutions which constitute their potential. These include:

- a centralised command system based on service hierarchy taking into account ranks and service positions while maintaining a high level of service discipline;
- a developed military infrastructure and constantly supplemented and modernised personnel, technical and material potential;
- multidimensional mobility with the use of military logistic systems allowing to undertake actions even in the most unfavourable conditions in any place in the world;

DOI: 10.4324/9781003353812-8

- an independent system of training and professional development of soldiers carried out by entities belonging to the armed forces;
- legal and organisational solutions allowing for internal control and elimination of problems in the functioning of the armed forces;
- maintaining combat readiness, which in practice means the ability to take immediate action in a situation of emergency or other events requiring an organised response of formations responsible for security (national, internal).

Contemporary challenges to be addressed by the armed forces are not limited to actions of military nature. In fact, all contemporary security strategies of the European Union member states contain guidelines relevant to the armed forces taking actions of non-military character as well. In the case of the occurrence of specific threats requiring the intervention of organised military forces, they are an indispensable element of the actions taken, the best example of which were the initiatives implemented by the army within the framework of the fight against the COVID-19 pandemic.

## 7.1 Problems and threats for the armed forces in the event of a pandemic

For centuries, the existence of armed forces was based primarily on military potential and the ability to use it in both offensive and defensive military operations. The development of societies, the progressing industrial revolution and the technical development in all aspects of modern life are the reasons why the use of the capabilities of military technology and the resources of the armed forces increasingly often bears the hallmarks of strictly non-military activities. Military logistics and other specialised elements of particular types of troops, which are part of every modern armed forces, are formed and managed in a way making it possible to both fulfil military tasks and directly support civil authorities in various non-military operations. Such utilitarianism in the use of armed forces is one of the pillars of contemporary military alliances, with civil-military cooperation playing a role in supporting peace as well (Zupančič, 2015).

The North Atlantic Treaty Organisation (NATO), which is perceived as the greatest guarantor of security and peace in the world, includes in its strategy the need to use the military potential of the member states for activities supporting civil authorities in crisis situations (Ministerial, 1998).

Armed forces around the world carry out their role in supporting civilian actors within the framework of specialised civil-military cooperation (CIMIC). The main objective of this type of activity is to support the military mission by establishing and maintaining cooperation with civilian actors in the area of military operation. The armed forces deploy soldiers with special training and extensive experience acquired through many years of service in conflict areas to establish relations with the civilian population, local authorities and other entities representing the interests of the local community.

Armed forces, when taking action in the civil-military area, follow several fundamental principles, which include:

- the principle of cultural awareness, which consists in understanding and respecting local history, traditions, the culture of a given community, local customs and, very importantly, the applicable law;
- the principle of common purpose, which consists in maintaining and constantly reinforcing the established cooperation, advice on how to achieve the objectives of the mission offered to commanders of military units stationed in areas covered by CIMIC operations;
- the principle of bilateral responsibility, which is based on a clear delimitation of the scope of cooperation with the civilian side, which defines the areas of responsibility and roles of the respective parties;
- the principle of civilian benefits, which is to identify opportunities for tangible benefits in civil-military cooperation. Within this principle, it is important to define the needs and expectations of the civilian side in relation to the military;
- the principle of obtaining an explicit agreement from the civilian side on the conduct of CIMIC activities;
- the principle of transparency of proceedings, based on an atmosphere of trust through the conduct of concrete and overt acts by the armed forces;
- the principle of effective communication through regular, open and direct contacts (Padányi, 2019).

The execution of tasks by the armed forces during CIMIC cooperation requires the use of several organisational components, including:

- a conceptual component, which defines the policy of actions, their planning based on relevant guidelines and accepted operational procedures, as well as supervision and coordination of civil-military cooperation during both exercises and specific operations;
- a training and education component, which provides courses, training and refresher courses and other useful forms of professional preparation of soldiers and civilians to achieve optimum levels of cooperation in CIMIC operations;
- an adequate and efficient organisational structure.

Thanks to the above-mentioned principles of operation and organisational components forming the foundations of civil-military cooperation, it is possible to achieve three basic functions of CIMIC, i.e.:

- a liaison function, manifested by constant contact of the civilian environment cooperating with a military contingent;

- a civil support function (assistance to civil authorities, social organisations and the local population) by the military contingent;
- a civilian support function to military operations carried out by the armed forces.

The experience gained as part of the CIMIC missions, made it possible to identify many needs and areas of civil-military cooperation. For this reason, activities involving the development of the civil-military interactions (CMI) doctrine have been launched within NATO since May 2014 (Van Koeveringe, 2016). Under peacetime conditions, armed forces support civilian authorities by directing for cooperation not only CIMIC specialists but also soldiers of other specialisations, including bomb disposal experts, logisticians, communications and IT specialists, military medical personnel, military chemists or specialists in combating biological and chemical threats, and military transport aviation crews. The CMI doctrine covers a wide group of initiatives based on communication, planning and coordination of undertakings carried out by bodies and units belonging to the NATO alliance together with various types of civilian entities and institutions. The aim of activities carried out within the framework of CMI doctrine is to increase the effectiveness of multifaceted initiatives and raise the level of efficiency of responding to emergent crisis situations of non-military character.

CIMIC as well as CMI partnerships have been created with activities of the armed forces as part of foreign missions in mind, but many years of experience gained as a result of the implementation of this type of operations of non-military character allow for more effective use of the possessed pro-civilian military potential. This is extremely important in the context of responding to crisis situations, the best example of which were the challenges faced by the armed forces during the COVID-19 pandemic.

The actions taken to control the COVID-19 pandemic by the armed forces of the member states of the NATO alliance once again demonstrated that the military component is an indispensable element of an effective response to crisis situations in the modern world. In documents published by the European Parliament, among others, it was stated that in the context of the COVID-19 pandemic, both the scale and scope of non-military actions carried out by NATO armed forces were on an unprecedented scale (Latici, 2020). Of course, before the outbreak of the pandemic, the alliance had conducted many humanitarian, rescue and aid operations in many parts of the world, but these were mostly local or regional operations with limited personnel and technical resources.

Together with NATO's actions taken in relation to the COVID-19 pandemic, problems and threats which the Alliance had to face also emerged. In an attempt to systematise these problems, two main categories can be identified: organisational problems and legislative and information problems.

Organisational problems, which not only NATO had to cope with in the fight against the COVID-19 pandemic, include interdependence in the supply chain in today's global supply market. The economic benefits of globalisation and delocation are also a threat of some kind, especially with the distorted diversification of supply. For more than ten years now, Western countries' dependence on Chinese imports has increased significantly in many areas that are also important for the defence sector. Examples in this regard include supplies for the EU and US electronics producers, for the sector using rare earth elements, and also supplies of essential components for European producers of semiconductors and medical materials (Garcia-Herrero et al., 2020).

The spread of the pandemic meant that over 30% of all NATO training and advisory activities in 2020 were significantly reduced, re-modelled or even postponed. There was an 80% reduction in the number of military personnel carrying out these activities, which was intended to minimise potential threats to the Alliance's operational readiness, including the rapid reaction force (De Maio, 2020). It became a priority for the Alliance to ensure the health (epidemiological) safety of soldiers, especially in the case of field exercises with the participation of international military components. NATO actions were based on the protocol for hybrid threats (Rynning, 2020). The Alliance, maintaining a high level of operational readiness, focused on ensuring resilience and continuity of activities carried out within the framework of its missions, training and exercises. Large military manoeuvres such as BALTOPS (Baltic Sea exercises) with the participation of Alliance member states were reorganised (only separated air and sea components were used) to satisfactorily achieve operational objectives while minimising the epidemiological threat (Eckstein, 2020). Of course, the full testing of the military components and the achievement of a high level of synergy in military operations were out of the question.

The rapid pace of the pandemic and its global impact meant that the Alliance had to respond flexibly and quickly to emerging and COVID-19-related challenges by, among other things, expanding the Euro-Atlantic Disaster Response Coordination Center (EADRCC) in terms of personnel and technology. The Center operates on a 24/7 basis at NATO Headquarters and plays the role of a point of information exchange and coordination of the response by NATO member states and partner countries in the event of a disaster in the Euro-Atlantic area. While previous NATO rescue and assistance operations, for example, in Afghanistan or after Hurricane Katrina in the US, did not require significant strengthening of the EADRCC, the COVID-19 pandemic forced a rapid reorganisation of the Alliance's structures to enable multifaceted operations allowing coordination of logistical assistance and rescue activities. During the logistics and transport activities the already proven solutions based on the activities of NATO's Support and Procurement Agency (NSPA) were used. The Agency has been responsible since 1958 for, among other things, the logistics of the Alliance's military air transport, the purchase of equipment necessary for humanitarian missions and the provision of medical services worldwide by NATO military components. NATO's logistics operations also benefited from the Strategic Airlift International Solution (SALIS) and the Strategic Airlift Capability (SAC) mechanisms used since the early 20th century. These enabled the rapid delivery of medicines and medical equipment, as well as field hospitals to requesting Alliance countries, and confirmed NATO's reliable relationships with the private sector (NATO's, 2021).

The legislative and information problems, manifested by the non-syn-chronous implementation of NATO's actions in the fight against the COVID-19 pandemic, included, above all, the different perceptions (especially in February 2020) of the threat posed by the pandemic by politicians representing the leading countries in the Alliance and by the NATO Secretary General. While the virus was already killing on a massive scale in Italy, the threat from the pandemic, among others, continued to be downplayed in the US. Even in the annual report published on 19 March 2020, which contains a review of NATO's activities for the previous year, when the epidemiological situation in European countries was already very bad, the sections of the report devoted to the Alliance's future activities, i.e. investing in security or modernising NATO, did not include any information relating to the most serious challenges posed by the pandemic (Stoltenberg, 2020). The Alliance took its first real action at the end of March 2020 by sending a shipment of medical equipment from South Korea and China to Romania, the Czech Republic and Slovakia, among other places (Kelement, 2020). In the following months, the Alliance's assistance, coordinated by the EADRCC, took on a global character.

In the V4 countries, a strong response to the spread of the pandemic took place in mid-March 2020. In Poland, the first case of coronavirus infection was confirmed on 4 March and a state of epidemic emergency was introduced on 14 March (Regulation of the Minister of Health of 13 March 2020). In Slovakia, the first case of coronavirus was confirmed on 6 March, a national emergency was declared on 12 March and a state of emergency was declared by the Slovakian government from 16 March (Uznesenie Vlády Slovenskej Republiky č. 114 z 15. marca, 2020). In the Czech Republic, three cases of coronavirus were confirmed on 1 March and a state of emergency was declared on 12 March (Usnesení vlády České, 2020). In Hungary, the first case of infection was confirmed on 4 March and a state of emergency was introduced on 11 March.[1]

In all V4 countries, practically from the beginning of the introduction of extraordinary measures or even earlier, the armed forces of these countries participated in rescue and assistance operations. In Poland, as early as February, aircraft from the 8th Base of Transport Aviation were used to transport Poles from China back home (gov.pl/web/obrona 2021). In March and early April, the air force of the Slovak Republic provided medical equipment and supplies for Slovak soldiers serving on NATO peacekeeping missions in Bosnia and Herzegovina, and also transported home Slovaks working in Scotland and the UK (https://www.mosr 2021). The medical personnel of the armed forces of the Czech Republic have already taken intensive measures, including strengthening the services of the National Integrated Rescue System, since 10 March 2020. Czech military doctors and paramedics carried out, among other things, health checks on people crossing borders and the military aviation personnel delivered coronavirus test packs from China (https://www.mocr.2021). The Hungarian armed forces undertook the first operations codenamed Corridor on 12 March on the M1, M5 and M7 motorways, where military gendarmerie together with the police patrolled designated rest areas for travellers returning to the country or transiting through Hungary.

Countering disinformation activities was another threat that the services belonging to the Alliance had to deal with in the fight against the COVID-19 pandemic. The most active in spreading false information and conspiracy theories against NATO were the secret services of Russia and China. The actions of these two countries have attempted to discredit the Alliance and its actions, and in some cases have even tried to blame the Alliance's armed forces for spreading the virus (Ozawa, 2020). In response to the accusations and intensification of fake news, NATO's Public Diplomacy Division was expanded, which monitored media reports on an ongoing basis and responded to all false information in cooperation with the European Union institutions. One effective instrument in combating disinformation was the creation of a website "NATO-Russia: setting the records straight", on which the Alliance's position on false reports appearing in the Russian-language media was regularly published. The Public Diplomacy Division worked closely with the EU's European External Action Service (EEAS) in its efforts to neutralise disinformation activity by Russia and China. In the near future, a specialised service for combating disinformation must be created within the NATO structures, capable of immediately counteracting any hostile manifestations of international military propaganda. This service will be able to identify disinformation threats in real time, verify and debunk false information about the actions of the Alliance and provide training for NATO soldiers and services in responding to information warfare threats. As part of this activity, the Alliance needs to strengthen cooperation with the European Union (East, 2021).

The dynamic development of the COVID-19 pandemic, which in a very short time assumed a global dimension, has highlighted the lack of a protocol containing algorithms for the conduct of NATO components in terms of maintaining continuity of statutorily implemented activities in the event of such crises. The Alliance demonstrated its ability to adapt quickly and maintain an acceptable operational level as regards stabilisation, peacekeeping and training missions. Unfortunately, this was an action-reaction approach based more on the rules that are the pillars of NATO's functioning, and lacking detailed, pre-tested guidelines containing precise models for action in the event of a global, epidemiological threat. Among the shortcomings of an organisational nature, in the context of protecting the Alliance's basic operational capabilities, one should point out the lack of mechanisms ensuring epidemiological protection (lack of protective and preventive vaccinations) for NATO staff of rapid reaction units. As a result, the soldiers and personnel of the alliance taking emergency action in connection with the pandemic were not adequately immunoprotected (De Maio, 2020).

On the basis of NATO's experience gained during the COVID-19 pandemic, the above-described threats to the functioning of the armed forces are only some of the potential problems which will have to be addressed in the future by the states forming not only this military alliance. In practice, the catalogue of threats of non-military character will always be open, as a consequence of the constant evolution of social life on all continents and the technological progress that the whole modern world has experienced.

## 7.2 NATO's response to the pandemic

The NATO Alliance in taking action related to the COVID-19 pandemic adopted two parallel levels of response. First of all, the continuity of the ongoing stabilisation, humanitarian and peacekeeping operations and missions was ensured while raising the level of health safety for personnel and soldiers of the Alliance countries performing tasks within the framework of these operations. One of the applied solutions was to modify or limit ongoing exercises using separated military components such as the air force or navy. These decisions were taken at the end of March 2020 on the basis of internal consultations among Alliance members, and other solutions were also adopted as part of the NATO Defence Ministers' meeting in June of that year to prepare the Alliance for the second wave of the COVID-19 pandemic.

In response to the first wave of the pandemic, the EADRCC initiated in March 2020 the delivery of medical supplies and materials that went to Romania, Poland and Moldova, among others, and NATO forces forming the KFOR military component in Kosovo supported 14 Kosovo municipalities in April with the donation of clothing, food, and protective and medical equipment for Kosovo health system personnel. A total of 17 missions were carried out in 2020 using the SALIS mechanism, providing 950 tonnes of medical supplies and equipment (Stoltenberg, 2020). Unfortunately, the actions taken were not always free of errors. Lack of due diligence in the quality control of the equipment imported as part of the aid operations from China or Russia resulted, for example, in Italy receiving completely useless equipment and decontamination agents. At the same time, the countries supplying this defective equipment, which had been portraying themselves as leaders in international humanitarian aid in the wake of the COVID-19 pandemic, took over the information space using the global corona crisis in their propaganda campaigns. According to the former Commander-in-Chief of NATO in Europe, General Ben Hodges, the Alliance did not properly recognise the elements of information warfare introduced under the banner of humanitarian aid by China and Russia into the world news services (Wesel, 2020).

Within the structures of the alliance, the COVID-19 Task Force was established at the Supreme Headquarters Allied Powers Europe (SHAPE) in

Mons (Belgium), whose task was to coordinate the provision of medical aid not only for NATO member states, but also for the countries covered by stabilisation divisions, and for the countries which requested such aid from the international community. The Alliance, using its logistic capabilities in cooperation with the armed forces of member states, carried out, among others, transport of patients, medicines, disinfectants, military medical staff, medical equipment in the form of military field hospitals, respirators or equipment for individual epidemiological protection of medical staff, food distribution. Soldiers forming part of NATO's rapid response military components carried out disinfection of public spaces, assisted with COVID-19 testing and provided expert psychological support to vulnerable people. In addition, support was provided to local health systems in areas where the Alliance forces were operating, for example, in Afghanistan or Iraq. In the actions taken against the first wave of the COVID-19 pandemic by the armed forces of the Alliance countries, a total of more than 500,000 soldiers and military personnel participated in supporting civilian authorities, as part of which NATO carried out, in addition to the above SALIS transports, among others, 350 flights with medical personnel, transported more than 1,500 tonnes of medical equipment using military equipment and built more than 100 field hospitals with 25,000 beds under a special sanitary regime (Stoltenberg, 2020).

As part of the NATO Science & Technology Organisation mechanism, in April 2020, NATO Chief Scientist Dr Bryan Wells activated the Alliance's scientific network of more than 6,000 experts to address the most pressing issues related to the functioning of the Alliance's armed forces during and after the pandemic, including but not limited to effective methods of virus detection and raising situational awareness of pandemic risks or solutions to enhance immunity in the future (after the COVID-19 pandemic).

The research effort allowed the identification of the main directions for the implementation of scientific cooperation, which were specified in six main categories:

- research to better understand disinformation activities about the pandemic and how to effectively counter disinformation;
- research on eliminating health risks to military personnel during post-pandemic relief operations;
- research on the use of analytical tools by scientists from the NATO network of experts to plan the Alliance's response during potential future pandemics;
- research focused on better use of modern technology for training military commanders in charge of pandemic relief operations;
- research on analyses and lessons learned from COVID-19 pandemic operations for the national defence systems of the Alliance member states;
- research on the ethical dimensions of support in the Alliance's military pandemic relief operations (Mesterhazy, 2020).

In 2020, NATO's Science for Peace and Security Programme also launched research or adopted existing solutions, including:

- the COVID-19 rapid diagnostics project was initiated, in which scientists from Switzerland supported mobile analytical laboratories in Morocco and Tunisia with their expertise;
- a project to develop new tools for rapid and accurate diagnosis of SARS-CoV-2 infection was launched involving scientists from Italy's Istituto Superiore di Sanità (National Health Institute) and Tor Vergata University Hospital, together with the University Hospital of Basel University in Switzerland. In this 24-month research initiative, through a multidisciplinary approach, experts in immunology, virology and molecular biology aim to develop solutions to increase the speed and efficiency of the virus diagnosis (https://www.esteri 2021);
- an existing solution called Adapting the Next-Generation Incident Command System was used, in which researchers at the Massachusetts Institute of Technology (MIT) in the US developed a systemic IT tool for managing forest fires in California and Australia. This system is being implemented in the Western Balkans and has been used by, among others, North Macedonia to combat the COVID-19 pandemic. The system enables inter-institutional and international cooperation in the event of a crisis situation. It allows, among other things, the exchange of information, maps, videos and photos in real time among the participants of rescue operations.
- the NOCOVID project, within which organisational and technological solutions enabling rapid, mobile and large-scale diagnostics of epidemiological threats with particular regard to coronavirus were created. The results of this project were implemented in Moldova, Morocco and Tunisia (Stoltenberg, 2020).

The information policy of the Alliance regarding the presentation of the results of the scientific research undertaken on the COVID-19 pandemic is very parsimonious, as in the published documents and reports one can find only information indicating the initiation of scientific cooperation, but no data on the acquired results of this research. As indicated in the information on the website administered by NATO, the results of the studies initiated in 2020, which on average take two years, are to be published and presented to the public.[2]

With regard to the exchange of experiences of medical personnel in the fight against COVID-19, the Alliance cooperated with the European Union under the mechanism of The Multinational Medical Coordination Center/ European Medical Command (MMCC/EMC). The aim of these activities was to increase the level of readiness and capabilities of NATO medical services through closer cooperation with the civilian health systems of the European Union member states (Lange, 2020).

In the initial phase of the fight against the pandemic (spring 2020), NATO carried out more than a hundred military transports with essential assistance. Airlifts included field hospitals with complete equipment, medical equipment including respirators, medical oxygen cylinders, personal protective equipment, hazmat suits, masks and protective gloves, surgical gowns and medical supplies such as injection needles and syringes necessary for COVID-19 vaccinations, supplies and equipment necessary for room disinfection, COVID-19 test kits, medicines and food. Assistance was directed to countries such as Italy, Spain, Albania, Bosnia and Herzegovina, Colombia, Georgia, Moldova, Montenegro, North Macedonia, Slovenia, Serbia, Czech Republic, Slovakia, the UK, Luxembourg and Ukraine, among others.

The Alliance used its special forces and international operational components as part of its efforts. These are the already mentioned EADRCC and the NATO Support and Procurement Agency (NSPA) Southern Operational Centre in Taranto (Italy) and the NATO Rapid Deployable Corps Italy (NRDC-ITA) based in Milan. NRDC is an international component of NATO that has an immediate mobilisation capability to provide the necessary assistance to respond to emergencies on the territory of the Alliance member states or anywhere on the ground. NRDC supported local authorities in the Italian region of Lombardy, which was one of the most affected EU territories, during the initial period of the fight against the pandemic. The V4 countries, as part of the action taken by the EADRCC, NSPA and NRDC, received assistance in the form of:

- transport of medical equipment (ventilators, personal protective equipment, COVID-19 tests, medicines, equipment for field hospitals);
- support for the treatment of virus-infected and tested persons, assisted by military medical personnel from the armed forces of NATO member states; support in the decontamination of national health system facilities (Ištok, 2020).

In June 2020, the NATO Pandemic Response Trust Fund was established with an initial capital of EUR 5 million, which was supported by sixteen Alliance member states, including the V4 countries. The financial aid was used to create medical aid packages (medical equipment, supplies, field hospitals), which were transferred to the countries most affected by the pandemic, such as Bosnia and Herzegovina, Iraq, the Republic of Moldova, Tunisia and Ukraine.

As part of the ongoing efforts to combat the COVID-19 pandemic, the NATO Alliance worked closely with other international organisations, including the European Union, the United Nations Office for the Coordination of Humanitarian Affairs (UN OCHA), the World Health Organisation (WHO) and the United Nations World Food Programme.

NATO's cooperation with the EU was mainly based on the exchange of experience and best practices in the field of, inter alia, the application of risk assessment procedures, the use of research instruments enabling the assessment of the degree of immunity of personnel, the implementation of medical evacuation procedures and countering hybrid threats, as well as responding to situations with a large number of victims, the occurrence of collective panic or the protection of critical infrastructure. Regular contacts between NATO and the EU were maintained at the working level in the form of regular briefings between the EADRCC and the EU's Emergency Response Coordination Centre (ERCC) and between the NATO COVID-19 Task Force and the one created by the EU's European External Action Service (EEAS) (Interview, 2021).

NATO launched a mechanism called Rapid Air Mobility on 31 March 2020, which involved the deployment of military aviation equipment and personnel to several EU countries. This was intended to ensure rapid air mobility and support Alliance partners in the delivery of seamless airlift of medical supplies across Europe. To this end, cooperation was undertaken with the European Organisation for the Safety of Air Navigation (EUROCONTROL), within which procedures were simplified for military transport flights by using NATO's unique call sign to speed up and better coordinate international flights, and checks and diplomatic briefings were shortened.[3]

The cooperation of the EADRCC with the UN and WHO consisted, among others, in joint coordination of activities in providing humanitarian and medical assistance in the areas where NATO forces operate within the framework of stabilisation and peacekeeping missions. Moreover, the aforementioned organisations also cooperate in the field of:

- providing necessary assistance in case of natural or human-initiated disasters in the areas covered by the UN and WHO humanitarian assistance;
- organisation of crisis management field exercises, which are carried out once a year by the EADRCC;
- organisation of seminars to discuss lessons learned from NATO, the UN and WHO coordinated emergency response operations.[4]

## 7.3 Legal regulations specifying operations of the armed forces in situations of epidemiological threats in Poland, the Czech Republic, Slovakia and Hungary

The effectiveness of actions taken by the armed forces in response to crisis situations depends on several factors. Undoubtedly, the most important determinants include legal regulations, which comprehensibly and exhaustively define the areas of activities and their scope reserved for the military as part of, among others, responding to non-military, including epidemiological, threats.

Undoubtedly, in the Visegrad Group (hereinafter: V4) made up of four Central European countries, i.e. Poland, the Czech Republic, Slovakia and

Hungary, the most important legal acts allowing for the involvement of the armed forces in the fight against the COVID-19 pandemic are the constitutions of these countries. They contain general dispositions regarding extraordinary measures in a form of organised actions by the state apparatus to counteract specific threats (e.g. a state of emergency, a state of natural disaster, martial law), if ordinary constitutional measures prove insufficient.

In the V4 countries, the description of the nature and scope of actions taken by, for example, rescue services, police or armed forces in connection with the occurrence of extraordinary measures is contained in laws and lower-level regulations (e.g. regulations, orders). Furthermore, the details of the implementation of rescue and relief actions are regulated by resolutions of the council of ministers and other executive authorities, the legislative authority (e.g. the president, the parliament), including ministries responsible for security (national, internal), healthcare or environmental protection.

In Poland, during a state of natural disaster, the armed forces support local state administration bodies (regional governors and local governments) in accordance with, inter alia, Article 18 of the Act of 18 April 2002 on the state of natural disaster (Ustawa z dnia 18 kwietnia 2002 r. o stanie klęski żywiołowej). The condition for the armed forces to be put in operation is the lack of possibility for the threat to be eliminated by civilian rescue services, with the actions by the military being restricted exclusively to the area covered by a given natural disaster. The soldiers remain under the command of their service superiors and perform tasks specified by the regional governor.

On the territory of the Slovak Republic, the use of the military component in rescue operations in connection with the occurrence of a state of natural disaster is possible on the basis of Articles 4 and 5 of Act No. 227 of 11 April 2002 on State security in the time of war, martial law, state of emergency and state of natural disaster and on the basis of paragraph 4 (2 and 4) of the Act No. 321 of 23 May 2002 on the Armed Forces of the Slovak Republic (Ustawa nr 227 z dnia 11 kwietnia 2002 r. o bezpieczeństwie państwa w czasie wojny). In their operations, the Slovak armed forces fully cooperate with the local state administration and local governments.

The Czech armed forces undertake rescue actions in connection with the occurrence of an emergency situation such as a state of natural disaster based, inter alia, on regulations arising from paragraph 9 (1-5) of the Act No. 240 of 28 June 2000 on crisis management (Ustawa nr 240 z dnia 28 czerwca 2000 r. o zarządzaniu kryzysowym).

The basis for the actions of the Hungarian armed forces in the event of a state of natural disaster is Article 8(3h) and Article 48(1b and 4) of the Hungarian Constitution of 25 April 2011 (Konstytucja Węgier z dnia 25 kwietnia r, 2011). The Czech and Hungarian soldiers undertake rescue and relief operations under the coordination of central and voivodship emergency headquarters and in close cooperation with local authorities.

In operations undertaken by the armed forces in the V4 member states, in connection with combating threats of non-military nature, such as natural disasters, epidemics, catastrophes, legal regulations governing the functioning of these formations or state rescue systems also apply. It would be impossible to list here all the legal acts at the rank of a statute, which define the organisation and functioning of uniformed services and forces or the organisation of individual rescue systems from Poland, the Czech Republic, Slovakia and Hungary, because the list would contain more than 50 such regulations.

For many years, the NATO Alliance, including the armed forces of the V4 countries, has been improving its activities carried out as part of non-military missions. In order for the effectiveness of these activities to reach a satisfactory level, it is necessary not only to develop human resources and modernise the military technical potential but also to amend and enact legal acts adequate to the development of "civil" threats, which constitute a clear indicator for conduct not only in the national arena but also, as demonstrated by the COVID-19 pandemic, in a global dimension.

## 7.4 The use of armed forces of Slovakia, Poland, Hungary and the Czech Republic in the fight against the COVID-19 pandemic – a comparative study

The involvement of the armed forces of the Visegrad Group countries in the fight against the COVID-19 pandemic provided important support to health systems and helped to bring the epidemiological situation under control in these countries. In the first year of the pandemic, supporting other state institutions, the armed forces of Slovakia, Poland, Hungary and the Czech Republic implemented basically the same four main types of activities on their own territory. These were activities involving medical support, logistics, support of other state and local government rescue or police services and implementation of other projects directly or indirectly related to the strategy to contain the spread of the pandemic and limit its health and socio-economic consequences.

As part of actions undertaken by the Polish Armed Forces, the Military Task Groups were established in all regions, whose role was to support the national health service in the framework of the national crisis management system. The actions of the Polish Armed Forces were conducted as part of two military operations under the codenames: Odporna Wiosna (Immune Spring) and Trwała Odporność (Permanent Immunity).

The aim of the Immune Spring operation was to mitigate the effects of the pandemic and to strengthen the resilience of local communities to the crisis. The operation provided support, at the request of the relevant sanitary authority or local government body. In contrast, Permanent Immunity operation focused on five types of action, i.e. prevention, identification, isolation, support and restoration. Unlike the former large-scale operation, the latter focused mainly on extinguishing outbreaks of coronavirus and activities were directed at supporting healthcare, sanitation services, local governments and regional governors in such a way as to neutralise the transmission of SARS-CoV-2. The nature of the activities was more relational, oriented towards point assistance in places that lost the ability to effectively fight the coronavirus, including through support for the national healthcare system and other institutions and maintaining readiness to support state emergency services and local governments in the area of non-military emergency activities.

In the fight against the first wave of the pandemic, about 9,000 soldiers representing various types of the Polish Armed Forces were deployed (The Polish Armed, 2021). Taking into account the current personnel and technical potential of the Polish Armed Forces, consisting of over 135,000 soldiers (Kowalczyk & Błaszczak, 2021), the size of the military component assigned at that time to combat the pandemic was not optimal.

The scope of tasks entrusted to individual types of the Polish Armed Forces in the two operations was very broad and included both the protection of the state borders together with the border guard, conducting jointly with the police activities for security and public order in the form of patrols aimed at controlling the observance of quarantine by the society, transport of food and personal protection equipment, delivery of food and medicines to persons in quarantine and groups particularly vulnerable to infection, delivery of protective equipment for medical personnel of district hospitals throughout the country in the form of, inter alia, hazmat suits, visors, shoe protectors, disinfectant fluids, thermometers, respirators, distribution of oxygen cylinders, care for veterans and families of medics (tasks were carried out by soldiers of the Territorial Defence Forces), care for residents of nursing homes (tasks were carried out by soldiers of the Territorial Defence Forces), carrying out tests for COVID-19, among others, in mobile swabs collection points (tasks were carried out by personnel and soldiers from the Centre for Diagnostics and Combating Biological Threats of the Military Institute of Hygiene and Epidemiology located in Puławy); evacuation by air of citizens of the Republic of Poland who, due to the global lockdown, could not reach the country on their own, and transport by air of personal protective equipment, decontamination of facilities, rooms, equipment and means of transport, construction of a container field hospital, mobile field laboratories, field emergency rooms and field decontamination points.

In addition to equipment available to individual types of troops belonging to the Polish Armed Forces, 14 military hospitals and 5 preventive medicine centres were also used in the fight against the pandemic. As part of the activities related to the second wave of the COVID-19 pandemic, 20,000 soldiers and military civilian personnel were involved, which constituted less than 15% of the total number of the Polish Armed Forces.[5]

The Armed Forces of the Slovak Republic, which constitute the second (after the police corps) most numerous uniformed force in this country (The approximately..., 2020), played an important role in combatting the

COVID-19 pandemic in 2020. As part of a nationwide effort codenamed Corona, all Slovak uniformed forces performed tasks aimed at limiting the impact of the pandemic, which was the direct reason for declaring a state of natural disaster across the country. An operation centre was activated within the Slovak armed forces, which worked closely with the government's crisis headquarters and coordinated the implementation of rescue and sanitary-epidemiological activities throughout the country around the clock. As part of the Corona operation, soldiers together with officers of other uniformed forces carried out many activities under the four sub-operations codenamed: Karuzela (Carousel), Parasol (Umbrella), Kurier (Courier) and Wspólna Odpowiedzialność (Joint Responsibility).

The activities of the Umbrella sub-operation, in which 1,500 soldiers participated from mid-April to the end of May 2020 during the most intensive period, were aimed at supporting the police corps of the Slovak Republic in ensuring security and public order in Roma settlements that had been isolated from other settlements due to the worsening epidemiological situation on their territory. The peak of infections in these settlements was recorded in mid-April and the last collective quarantine linked to the complete isolation of the Roma settlement was completed on 30 May 2020. In addition to strictly policing activities, soldiers also supported the operation of field swab collection points and transported COVID-19 tests to laboratories.

The Carousel operation, in which more than 200 soldiers participated, involved the support of the national health system by military medical personnel under the Department of the Chief Medical Officer of the Armed Forces of the Slovak Republic. Among other things, Slovak soldiers in 177 Roma settlements collected swabs for examination and disinfected field emergency rooms. In addition, they carried out intensive information activities to defuse social tension caused, among other things, by rumours of deliberate infection of the inhabitants of these settlements in order to evict them from illegally occupied housing (Vitko, 2020). In addition to military doctors and paramedics and soldiers from the chemical company, military aviation and land forces personnel also participated in the operation, which had a help-and-rescue character and was coordinated by both the Department of the Chief Medical Officer of the Armed Forces and the Office of the Chief Sanitary Inspector of the Slovak Republic (Vitko, 2020).

As part of the Courier operation, the Slovak Armed Forces carried out logistic tasks including transporting fuel for equipment used in sanitary-epidemiological operations and transporting medical equipment and personal protective equipment, which arrived from abroad and were distributed throughout the country from central warehouses of state reserves.

The Joint Responsibility operation has been the largest logistical operation in the history of the Armed Forces of the Slovak Republic, with the Ministry of Defence supporting the Ministry of the Interior as well as provincial offices and local governments. Approximately 5,000 swab collection points were organised throughout the country as part of the nationwide testing of citizens for the SARS-CoV-2 virus. More than 5.3 million people were tested in the three phases of testing, representing 96% of the country's population (Prvé, 2021).

The Armed Forces of the Slovak Republic also conducted a number of other activities as part of the fight against the COVID-19 pandemic, for example, together with the police corps, soldiers from the land forces carried out public security tasks at border crossing points with the Czech Republic, Poland, Austria and Hungary, soldiers assisted with transports of medical supplies, food and state reserves organised by the police corps throughout the country, logistic units of the Slovak Armed Forces were responsible for the provisioning of three state quarantine centres and the distribution of drinking water in Roma settlements and, finally, soldiers from the military gendarmerie carried out tasks involving the physical and epidemiological protection of facilities important for the smooth functioning of government offices (Paulech, 2021).

In the most intense period of the fight against the COVID-19 pandemic in Slovakia, 8,000 soldiers participated in the operations, which constituted almost 60% of the number of the country's armed forces. The involvement of the Slovak armed forces in pandemic-related activities on such a significant scale was due to several factors. First of all, the decision to test the entire nation for the presence of the coronavirus generated the need to involve all available forces at the disposal of the state and local government uniformed services. In addition to soldiers, this action involved officers of the police corps, firefighters, municipal police officers under the authority of local government and members of state and community rescue organisations and, of course, personnel of the Slovak health system. In addition, the Slovak armed forces have the most modern and largest logistical potential, which was used for provisioning and transporting people, equipment and medicines not only within the country. Military facilities, where collective quarantine or redistribution points for medical equipment and medicines have been organised, were also used in the operations undertaken by the armed forces.

The involvement of the Armed Forces of the Czech Republic in the activities related to the COVID-19 pandemic was similar to that of Poland and Slovakia. Czech soldiers supported the National Integrated Protection System by cooperating with local state administration bodies and local government bodies. Activities of the armed forces in this area were locally coordinated by Voivodship Military Staffs and the whole activity was supervised by the General Command of the Armed Forces of the Czech Republic. In their actions, Czech soldiers used their extensive experience gained during many peacekeeping and stabilisation missions undertaken, inter alia, under the NATO mandate since 1999 (Pajer, 2013). In the fight against the pandemic, practically all types of troops forming the Czech armed forces carried out tasks of a logistical, preventive or technical nature together with other domestic and foreign institutions and services.

The Czech soldiers as part of operation Eye and operation Smart Quarantine supported the national healthcare system by carrying out the following activities:

- transporting by air tests and personal protective equipment and medical equipment for hospitals and health care facilities from other countries;
- together with the police, they carried out patrol and intervention tasks at border crossings involving enforcement of regulations connected with the dynamically changing epidemiological situation by persons crossing the country (among others, the tasks were carried out by soldiers from the 7th Mechanised Brigade in Hranice);
- military medical personnel controlled an average of 15,000 people per day at border crossings by, among other things, measuring body temperature and conducting a medical history;
- military medical personnel and student-soldiers from the Faculty of Medicine of the Defence University in Brno supported national hospitals and healthcare facilities where patients infected with SARS-CoV-2 were treated;
- throughout the country, military medical personnel and logistic services of the Czech Armed Forces organised swab collection points for testing (among others, the task was carried out by the 153rd Engineering Battalion in Olomouc);
- military logistic services were responsible for transporting medical supplies and equipment, medicines and other items necessary for combating the pandemic throughout the country. In the course of the operations, the soldiers closely cooperated with the Administration of State Material Reserves;
- the Czech Air Force also transported people involved in road accidents to hospitals, supporting the air rescue, which was overloaded with tasks related to the pandemic;
- soldiers from military gendarmerie protected facilities important for the proper functioning of government administration, including providing epidemiological protection and disinfection of these facilities;
- soldiers from special land units of the Czech Armed Forces served as drivers of Czech healthcare vehicles;
- logistic services and military medical personnel built a hospital, mobile field laboratories and field emergency rooms;
- land troops helped to care for residents of nursing homes (including soldiers from the Military Academy in Vyškov);
- soldiers from the units of reconnaissance and radio-electronic warfare support in Opava launched and operated call centres acting as telephone information points for persons in contact with the infected and providing emergency psychological aid (among others, such tasks were performed by soldiers from the 53rd Electronic Warfare Regiment in Opava);

in the initial phase of combatting the pandemic, civilian personnel and soldiers from logistic units, using their equipment and organising fundraising for the fabric, sewed protective masks and gloves for medical personnel and state service officers (among others, such activity was conducted by soldiers from the 533rd Drone Battalion in Prostejov);

as part of mobile teams, soldiers conducted tests for COVID-19 (including soldiers from 25th Missile and Air Defence Regiment in Strakonice);

scientists representing the Brno Defence University participated in research resulting in the production of more effective filters for protective masks for medical personnel dealing with the pandemic;

soldiers supported the Central Military Hospital in blood donation campaigns;

during the autumn 2020 elections for regional councils and the senate, the Czech Armed Forces together with the police secured polling stations to ensure public compliance with pandemic-related regulations. In addition, soldiers operated mobile voting stations known as drive-in, where people retrieved and cast their ballot papers directly from their cars.

During the fight against the first and second waves of the pandemic, the Czech Armed Forces repetitively deployed for action almost 15,000 soldiers. Soldiers from logistics units used more than 300 trucks, 80 smaller vehicles, 10 buses and also helicopters and transport aircraft belonging to the Czech Air Force every day.

The involvement of the Hungarian armed forces in activities related to the COVID-19 pandemic outbreak was quantitatively much smaller compared to the other V4 countries. As of 12 March 2020, a total of 900 soldiers and military police officers were deployed for police support activities at the southern border crossings. In pandemic-related prevention, protection and help and rescue activities, the most involved force was the Hungarian police with more than 40,000 officers. The military component played a supporting role in the actions taken by the uniformed services under the ministry of the interior.

On 14 March, the Hungarian government adopted Decision No. 1109/2020 on the establishment of Special Military Task Forces. Accordingly, the military were given the opportunity to interfere in many areas of the state administration, local government, as well as the country's economic sector. The minister of defence was obliged to provide a security umbrella for 140 state enterprises offering the so-called critical services in order to maintain their proper level of functioning. Assistance was provided to companies operating in the energy, telecommunications, transport and healthcare sectors. The armed forces helped, among others, the oil company MOL to protect transport corridors used for transporting liquid fuels. Together with police officers, soldiers also carried out activities at petrol stations consisting in controlling the observance of epidemiological restrictions by, among others, Romanian and Bulgarian citizens travelling from western European countries. Moreover, the Special Military Task Forces coordinated the return to the country of trucks belonging to the MOL concern, which got stuck on the territory of Italy (Informator, 2020). With the introduction of the curfew on 27 March 2020 by Government Decree No. 71/2020, the number of soldiers participating in prevention, patrol and intervention activities increased to 1,500.

The Government Decree No. 72/2020 of 28 March[6] established a system of security surveillance by the army and police over the operation of hospitals and medical supply warehouses. The minister of the interior was responsible for supervising the implementation of the tasks set by Decree No. 72 for Hungary's two largest uniformed forces. Army and police officers were appointed as Temporary Heads of Security Supervision of the state hospitals. By 18 April, the Hungarian armed forces had posted officers in 51 hospitals throughout the country. Their task was to protect transports with medical supplies, protect warehouses with medical equipment and supplies used in the fight against the pandemic and supervise the deployment and use of military equipment intended for activities including sanitary-epidemiological protection of hospital facilities. The delegated officers could not decide on any issues related to the provision of medical assistance offered in these hospitals (Informator, 2020).

Within the scope of their operations, the Hungarian armed forces also carried out similar tasks to the Polish and Czech armed forces under the state of emergency declared by the government, such as transport of equipment and personal protective equipment for medical personnel, as well as food and other donations obtained from nationwide collections for combating the pandemic, disinfection of nursing homes for the elderly and selected facilities where aid was provided to persons infected with the virus, construction of field screening points and health checkpoints at the entrances to government facilities and joint patrol and intervention actions with the police aimed at controlling citizens' compliance with sanitary and epidemiological regulations during the restrictions announced by the government. Administrative and logistical support was provided to 93 hospitals located throughout the country, and patrolling activities were reinforced at southern border crossings, where an additional 1,200 soldiers were deployed.

In addition, the Hungarian government, under NATO's security partnership mechanism, deployed 200 soldiers to support the nationwide testing of Slovak citizens for the SARS-CoV-2 virus. Since the beginning of their membership in NATO, Hungarian soldiers have always demonstrated above-average commitment to non-military rescue and assistance operations (Csiki, 2015).

As part of NATO's pandemic relief efforts, the V4 countries received support in the form of SALIS airlifts of medical supplies, ventilators and personal protective equipment for medical personnel. The Czech Republic also received support in the form of military medical personnel from Germany, the UK and the US, while Slovakia was supported in its pandemic efforts by military paramedics from Austria and the aforementioned Hungarians.

Summarising the research material used in the preparation of this chapter, it should be noted that unfortunately it does not exhaust all substantive aspects relating to the role played by both NATO and the armed forces of the Visegrad Group countries in the fight against the COVID-19 pandemic. This is mainly due to the fact that the involvement of soldiers in fighting the pandemic, which has not yet been finally resolved, continues uninterrupted. Moreover, the nature and magnitude of the actions undertaken by NATO and the V4 armed forces are constantly changing, which is the reason why a comprehensive summary of the role of the military component in the fight against the SARS-CoV-2 virus is still a long way off.

As can be seen from the analysis of the relevant literature, legal acts and media reports, the NATO Alliance fulfilled its tasks within its capabilities to support individual countries in activities preventing the spread of the pandemic. A number of mechanisms and organisational and logistical solutions currently available to NATO were activated, which has been reflected in real and effective assistance provided to NATO member states. The Alliance also provided humanitarian and material aid to other countries that had requested it. Within the framework of its operations against COVID-19, NATO carried out many tasks of logistical nature, including, above all, the transport of individual protective equipment for medical personnel and various types of medical equipment. The Alliance also initiated research activities aimed at obtaining effective immune protection against the virus, supported healthcare systems in many countries and also protected personnel carrying out activities as part of NATO military missions around the world.

The COVID-19 pandemic, which assumed a size and pace hitherto unknown in the modern world, was and continues to be a valuable lesson for, among others, all organisations providing humanitarian and medical assistance on a global scale. In its fight against the pandemic, NATO appears to have drawn on its many years of experience gathered around the world in non-military operations, and at the same time is an organisation capable of making flexible and rapid changes that improve the effectiveness of the Alliance. Undoubtedly, in this context, the main research hypothesis was confirmed. A certain shortcoming in the implementation of the Alliance's information policy should be considered as the lack of regularly published reports relating to NATO's activities for the civilian sector. Apart from promoting the Alliance, such studies would also allow us to draw useful information from the experience gained in this field.

As regards the auxiliary hypothesis which contained a partly critical view of the effectiveness of the Alliance's actions with the use of the established NATO Pandemic Response Trust Fund, it should be pointed out that, despite the delayed implementation of logistical assistance using the resources of the Fund, at least 16 countries received support during the first wave of infections, and the medical aid packages which were transferred (medical equipment, operational materials, field hospitals), the functioning of the healthcare systems in such countries as Bosnia and Herzegovina, Iraq or the Republic of Moldova, among others. However, one may have some doubts as to whether the funds of EUR 5 million collected within the framework of this Fund were sufficient in the context of the real needs generated by the pandemic and adequate to the financial capabilities of the sixteen countries subsidising the NATO Pandemic Response Trust Fund.

The second part of the auxiliary hypothesis, which assumed that in the Visegrad Group countries only units performing a supporting role for the main types of armed forces were deployed to fight the effects of COVID-19, has definitely not been confirmed, either. All V4 countries, as part of their efforts to slow down the pace of the pandemic and limit its socio-economic impact, used a wide range of their personnel and technical resources with varying intensity, making the armed forces play a key role in the fight against the pandemic especially in its initial phase. The experts who expressed their opinion on the place and role of the armed forces in the fight against the pandemic in the Visegrad countries unambiguously indicated that without the involvement of the potential of all types of troops forming the armies of these countries, an effective fight against the SARS-CoV-2 virus would not be possible. The participants of the expert interviews also took a position on the adopted research questions. The most important organisational and legal problems that may occur in connection with taking action by the armed forces of NATO member states in the event of a pandemic of a global nature included:

  in the organisational aspect, the lack of unanimity when implementing, on a global scale, the Alliance's actions requiring greater commitment of the resources held by the leading armies of the Alliance. This is due to the different ways in which NATO member states perceive the threats posed by a pandemic, especially in its initial phase;
  in the legal aspect, the lack of protocols and executive regulations accepted by the members of the Alliance, which would provide a basis for the implementation by the Alliance's Headquarters of immediate, targeted actions with the use of resources under the command of member states' armies, in the event of non-military crisis situations such as a pandemic or natural disasters of an international character.

According to experts, in terms of the technical challenges highlighted by the COVID-19 pandemic, NATO Command should significantly expand its science and research capacity in the coming years. Particular importance should be given to the Science for Peace and Security Programme, as part of the organisational structure of NATO Headquarters in a permanent form. Moreover, the technological and scientific-research potential used so far by NATO, in the form of centres such as the Center for Maritime Research and Experimentation located in La Spezia, Italy (CMRE), should also be directed towards the identification of threats of an epidemiological or biological nature, which will allow effective plans to be drawn up to counter this kind of threat.

The assistance of armed forces from NATO member states in the fight against COVID-19, which was the essence of the second research question, can be described, according to experts, as adequate to the development of the situation, optimal in terms of available capabilities and adapted to the international political situation that existed during the initial period of the pandemic. The SALIS and SAC mechanisms, verified in earlier NATO missions, allowed for the rapid supply of medicines and medical equipment, thus confirming the legitimacy of the Alliance's maintaining good relations with the private sector.

The rescue operations undertaken jointly by NATO and the European Union in connection with the pandemic, in the form of coordinated logistical operations, transport or the purchase of the necessary medical equipment, also pointed to the existence of certain discrepancies in the applied procedures. This area of cooperation between both international institutions has also highlighted the need to create common legislative solutions to facilitate faster action. The creation of a common warehouse on the territory of the European Union for both institutions, where equipment would be stored for immediate use in the event of a biological, epidemiological or chemical threat occurring in the EU, would also be worth considering.

In terms of the legal regulations in force in the V4 countries relating to responding to threats of an epidemiological nature, experts arrive at similar conclusions. In their opinion, the legal regulations in force in the V4 countries well define the role and tasks of the state administration, local governments and citizens in preventing and counteracting various types of crisis situations. There are some differences of opinion regarding the detailed regulation of responding to non-military threats in the constitution, as is the case in Hungary. According to some experts, the constitution should not contain overly detailed instructions and indications concerning, for example, the state's response to crisis situations but should only contain general directions of actions in this respect. Details should be covered by lower-ranking legal acts, such as statutes, which are much easier to amend. In the dynamically changing realities of socio-cultural life, with ever-increasing climate change and in connection with other threats related to the exploitation of the world's natural resources, this solution seems to be optimal.

The experts unequivocally indicated, as part of the answer to the question concerning the effectiveness of the actions taken by the armed forces of Slovakia, Poland, Hungary and the Czech Republic in the fight against SARS-CoV-2, that without the multifaceted and intensive (especially during the first wave of infections) involvement of the military component, the size and effects of the spread of the pandemic would have been even more severe for the societies of these countries. The personal and technical potential of modern armed forces is a driving power not only in terms of national defence but also in the sector of non-military activities in which soldiers are increasingly involved.

It is nowadays difficult to imagine the functioning of an independent and stable state without well-organised armed forces. With the collapse of the realities of the bipolar world, the role of the modern army has also changed. NATO, which guarantees in its doctrine not only collective defence but also humanitarian aid, is another determinant in the transformation of the armed forces of the EU states, including Poland, the Czech Republic, Slovakia and Hungary, as members of the Alliance. Through, among other things, modernisation of their equipment, raising the qualifications of military personnel and cooperation with other national services, as well as thanks to international cooperation, national military components are significantly increasing their usefulness in performing tasks for the benefit of broadly understood internal security, including epidemiological security, the best example of which was the activity of the armed forces of the V4 countries during the fight against the COVID-19 pandemic in 2020.

## Notes

1 https://www.origo.hu/itthon/percrolpercre/20200311-koronavirus-operativ-torzs-tajekoztato.html (accessed: 10 March 2021).
2 (https://www.nato 2021).
3 (https://www.nato 2021).
4 (https://www.nato 2021).
5 (https://www.wojsko 2021).
6 Informator (2020). Informator Parlamentu Węgier nr 23 z dnia 27 kwietnia 2020 r. pt. Zastosowanie armii w przeciwdziałaniu koronawirusowi (Hungarian Parliamentary Information Sheet No. 23 of 27 April 2020 on "The use of the army in countering coronavirus"), published by the Directorate of Public Collections and Public Education. Available from: https://www.parlament.hu/documents/10181/4464848/Infojegyzet_2020_23_hadsereg_koronavirus-jarvanyban.pdf/b6ad6867-0d0e-08c9-6462-b3bf336cff07?t=1587974484535, accessed: 14 June 2021.

## References

Csiki, T. (2015). Lessons learnt and unlearnt. Hungary's 15 years in NATO. In R. Czulda, & M. Madej (Eds.), *Newcomers no more? Contemporary NATO and the Future of the Enlargement from the Perspective of "Post-Cold War" Members*. International Relations Research Institute in Warsaw & Jagello 2000 – NATO Information Center in Prague (pp. 59–72). ISBN 978-83-62784-04-2

De Maio, G. (2020). *NATO's response to COVID-19: Lessons for resilience and readiness. Foreign Policy*, Brookings.

East (2021). *East Stratcom Task Force is an EEAS initiative that focuses on countering disinformation and highlighting EU activities in Eastern Europe.* Electronic source: https://euvsdisinfo.eu, accessed: 6 June 2021

Eckstein, M. (2020). BALTOPS 2020 Will Only Hold At-Sea Events With Ships Commanded from Shore. *USNI News*, 11 June 2020.

Garcia-Herrero, A., Wolff, G., Xu, J., Poitiers, N., Felbermayr, G., Langhammer, R., Liu, W.-H., & Sandkamp, A. (2020). *EU-China trade and investment relations in challenging times*. Directorate General for External Policies of the Union, PE 603.492, May 2020, p. 33. ISBN 978-92-846-6633-1

Informator (2020). Informator Parlamentu Węgier nr 23 z dnia 27 kwietnia 2020 r. pt. Zastosowanie armii w przeciwdziałaniu koronawirusowi (Hungarian Parliamentary Information Sheet No. 23 of 27 April 2020 on The use of the army in countering coronavirus), published by the Directorate of Public Collections and Public Education. Available from: https://www.parlament.hu/documents/10181/4464848/Infojegyzet_2020_23_hadsereg_koronavirus-jarvanyban.pdf/b6ad6867-0d0e-08c9-6462-b3bf336cff07?t=1587974484535, accessed: 14 June 2021.

Interview (2021). Interview with Mirosław Lipka from Civilian Planning and Conduct Capability European External Action Service (National Policy Expert & Police Expert in the Operations Division CPCC EEAS). The interview was conducted on 25 June 2021 in Brussel by Jacek Dworzecki

Ištok, D. (2020). *Koronavírus: SR žiada o pomoc NATO. Bude to lacnejšie a úplne transparentné, hovorí Naď* (Coronavirus: SR asks for NATO help. It will be cheaper and completely transparent, says Naď). Aktuality.sk, 1 Nov. 2020, Ringier Axel Springer Media s. r. o. Available from: https://www.aktuality.sk/clanok/836328/koronavirus-pomoc-nato-jaroslav-nad/, accessed: 17 May 2021.

Kelement, I. (2020). NATO zasahuje. Obrana, 5, Ministry of Defense of the Slovak Republic, p. 2, ISSN 1336-1910

Konstytucja Węgier z dnia 25 kwietnia 2011 r. (Urzędowy Organ Publikacyjny nr 43 z 2011 r. z późniejszymi zmianami). (The Constitution of Hungary of 25 April 2011. (Official Publication Authority No. 43 of 2011 as amended)

Kowalczyk, K., & Błaszczak, M. (2021). Polskie wojsko liczy 135 tys. żołnierzy razem z WOT. Bankier.pl, 3 March 2021. Available from: https://www.bankier.pl/wiadomosc/Blaszczak-Polskie-wojsko-liczy-135-tys-zolnierzy-razem-z-WOT-8066170.html, accessed: 19 May 2021

Lange, H. (2020). *...stay focused on achieving full operational capability of MMCC/EMC. European Military Medical Services*, 7 July, Beta Verlag und Marketing GmbH, pp. 5–7. Electronic source: https://military-medicine.com/article/4122-special-print-2020.html, accessed: 21 June 2021

Laţici, T. (2020). *NATO's response in the fight against coronavirus*. European Parliamentary Research Service, PE 651.955, June 2020, pp. 1–2

Ministerial (1998). *Ministerial Guidance for Civil Emergency Planning 1999-2000*. NATO, CEPD (IN V) (98) 24, 19 August 1998, p. 6

NATO's (2021). NATO's Response to the COVID-19 Pandemic. Factsheet, February, Public Diplomacy Division – Press & Media Section, pp. 1–4. Available from: www.nato.int/factsheets, accessed: 12 June 2021

Mesterhazy, A. (2020). The role of NATO's armed forces in the Covid-19 pandemic. Draft Special Report. NATO Defence and Security Committee, p. 6.

Ozawa, M. (2020). NATO and Russia in the time of Corona. Countering disinformation and supporting Allies. In T. Tardy (Ed.), *COVID-19: NATO in the Age of Pandemics* (pp. 21–30). NATO Defense College.

Padányi, J. (2019). The significance of civil-military cooperation in missions and mission preparation in crisis areas. In L. Ujházi, J. Kaló, & F. Petruska (Eds.), *Budapest report on Christian persecution* (p. 20). Háttér. ISBN 978-615-5124-67-9

Pajer, J. (Ed.) (2013). *Armed Forces of the Czech Republic a symbol of democracy and state sovereignty 1993-2012.* Ministry of Defence of the Czech Republic, pp. 95–121. ISBN 978-80-7278-601-5

Paulech, J. (2021). *How armed forces are dealing with the COVID-19 in Slovakia?,* Zväz Vojakov Slovenskej Republiky, pp. 1–9. Available from: http://euromil.org/wp-content/uploads/2020/04/COVID19_ZVSR.pdf, accessed: 25 February 2021

Prvé (2021). *Prvé kolo celoplošného testovania bolo úspešnou operáciou* (The first round of nationwide testing was a successful operation). Available from: http://www.minv.sk/?tlacove-spravy&sprava=prvekolo-celoplosneho-testovania-bolo-uspesnou-operaciou, accessed: 22 February 2021

Regulation of the Minister of Health of 13 March (2020). Rozporządzenie Ministra Zdrowia z dnia 13 marca 2020 r. w sprawie ogłoszenia na obszarze Rzeczypospolitej Polskiej stanu zagrożenia epidemicznego (Dziennik Ustaw z 2020 r., pozycja 4330); (Regulation of the Minister of Health of 13 March 2020 on the declaration of an epidemic threat in the territory of the Republic of Poland (Journal of Laws of 2020, item 4330)

Rynning, S. (2020). A renewed collective defense bargain? NATO in COVID's shadow. *NDC Policy Brief,* 16, pp. 1–4.

Stoltenberg, J. (2020). *The Secretary General's Annual Report 2019.* NATO, 19 March. Available from: https://www.nato.int/cps/en/natohq/opinions_174406.htm, accessed: 14 June 2021

The approximately (2020). The approximately 13,500-strong Armed Forces of the Slovak Republic include: Ground Forces, Air Force, Special Operations Forces, Military Police. Source: Defense and Security Market Report SLOVAKIA July 2020, prepared by EasyLink Business Services. Available from: https://exportvirginia.org/sites/default/files/2020-07/Slovakia_Defense_July2020.pdf, accessed: 7 Feb. 2021.

The Polish Armed (2021). The Polish Armed Forces include: Land Forces, Air Force, Navy, Territorial Defence Forces, Special Forces. Available from: https://www.wojsko-polskie.pl/rodzaje-szrp/, accessed: 11 February 2021

Uznesenie Vlády Slovenskej Republiky č. 114 z 15. marca 2020 k návrhu na vyhlásenie núdzového stavu podľa čl. 5 ústavného zákona č. 227/2002 Z. z. o bezpečnosti štátu v čase vojny, vojnového stavu, výnimočného stavu a núdzového stavu v znení neskorších predpisov, na uloženie pracovnej povinnosti na zabezpečenie výkonu zdravotnej starostlivosti a zakázanie uplatňovania práva na štrajk niektorým pracovníkom (Zbierka zákonov číslo 45 z 2020); (Resolution of the Government of the Slovak Republic no. 114 of 15 March 2020 on the proposal for a declaration of a state of emergency pursuant to Art. 5 of the Constitutional Act no. 227/2002 Coll. on the security of the state in time of war, state of war, state of emergency and state of emergency, as amended, to impose work duties on ensuring the provision of health care and prohibiting the exercise of the right to strike by certain workers (Collection of Laws No. 45 of 2020)

Usnesení vlády České (2020). Usnesení vlády České republiky o vyhlášení nouzového stavu pro území České republiky z důvodu ohrožení zdraví v souvislosti s prokázáním výskytu koronaviru /označovaný jako SARS CoV-2/ na území České republiky na dobu od 14.00 hodin dne 12. března 2020 na dobu 30 dnů (Sbírka zákonů Česká Republika 2020, částka 30, pozice 69); (Resolution of the Government of the Czech Republic on declaring a state of emergency for the territory of the Czech Republic due to health threats in connection with proving the occurrence of coronavirus /referred to as SARS CoV-2/ in the Czech Republic for 14.00 on 12 March 2020 for 30 days Czech Republic 2020, Vol. 30, Item 69)

Ustawa z dnia 18 kwietnia 2002 r. o stanie klęski żywiołowej (Dziennik Ustaw, 2002, Nr 62, pozycja 558 z późniejszymi zmianami). (Act of 18 April 2002 on the state of natural disasters (Journal of Laws, 2002, No. 62, item 558 as amended)

Ustawa nr 227 z dnia 11 kwietnia 2002 r. o bezpieczeństwie państwa w czasie wojny, stanu wojennego, stanu wyjątkowego i stanu klęski żywiołowej (Zbiór ustaw nr 97 z 2002 r. z późniejszymi zmianami); Ustawa nr 321 z dnia 23 maja 2002 r. o Siłach Zbrojnych Republiki Słowackiej (Zbiór ustaw nr 136 z 2002 r. z późniejszymi zmianami). [Act No. 227 of 11 April 2002 on State security during war, martial law, state of emergency and natural disaster (Collection of Acts No. 97 of 2002 as amended); Act No. 321 of 23 May 2002 on the Armed Forces of the Slovak Republic (Collection of Acts No. 136 of 2002 as amended)]

Ustawa nr 240 z dnia 28 czerwca 2000 r. o zarządzaniu kryzysowym (Zbiór Ustaw Republiki Czeskiej nr 73 z 2000 r. z późniejszymi zmianami). (Act No. 240 of 28 June 2000 on crisis management (Collection of Laws of the Czech Republic No. 73 of 2000 as amended)

Van Koeveringe, W. (2016). *Civil-military Cooperation and Military Police Interaction Status Report.* Hague: Civil-Military Cooperation Centre of Excellence, pp. 7–9.

Wesel, B. (2020). NATO pomaga w walce z koronawirusem (NATO is helping in the fight against coronavirus). Deutsche Welle, 4 April. Available from: https://www.dw.com/pl/nato-pomaga-w-walce-z-koronawirusem/a-53010578, accessed: 10 June 2021

Vitko, P. (2020). Operácia Karusel (Carousel operation). *Obrana*, May 2020, No. 5, Ministry of Defense of the Slovak Republic, pp. 4-5, ISSN 1336-1910

Zupančič, R. (2015). Civil-military cooperation in conflict and post-conflict zones: needed marriage also for small states? The case study of Slovenian Armed Forces in Kosovo and Afghanistan. *Journal of Slavic Military Studies*, 28, pp. 467–468. ISSN 1351-8046

# Summary

*Jolanta Itrich-Drabarek*

The fourth wave of the pandemic demonstrates the continuing helplessness of the countries of Central Europe in this matter. The pandemic of the unvaccinated, the scale of which could have been avoided, continues to have tragic consequences, but governments do not seem to have learnt their lesson.

The Visegrad Group countries, in addition to the problems associated with the SARS-CoV-2 pandemic, which are universal in nature, are characterised by a greater susceptibility to breaking and circumventing the law in force, because there is an increased number of irregularities and abuses of power associated with the previous level of socio-economic development, and governments, due to political connotations have a greater tendency to manage through restrictions, and the effects of the pandemic will be more profound than in other EU countries.

The situation within the Visegrad countries determined specific features of the politicisation of the pandemic. For example, in Poland, it took on the form of an umbrella syndrome, behind which the central government camouflaged the true purpose of its actions by introducing legal changes which violated the constitutional principles of presidential elections or the so-called abortion compromise, while in Slovakia, the government's crisis management policy became the main criterion for assessment of its efficiency and effectiveness and led to the resignation of the prime minister. Meanwhile, in Hungary, it exposed the main interest group, which is foreign capital, and the actions taken indicated that the stability of the internal government depends on its support, which was reflected in solutions promoting large companies and corporations.

The pandemic deepened the popularity of populists in Central Europe, who were able to use apparent methods (controlling and closing borders, building temporary hospitals, never mind that they were ill-equipped and overpaid) to strengthen and confirm their electorate in the belief that they were doing well, despite the fact that during the peak phase, around 700 people a day were dying in Poland. Despite the deaths of many people in the fourth wave of the pandemic, governments only semantically have vaccines to offer but, unfortunately, are unable to convince unvaccinated citizens to use them.

DOI: 10.4324/9781003353812-9

Activities to mitigate the effects of the SARS-CoV-2 pandemic are also undertaken at the sub-regional level. In the case of the analysed Visegrad Group (V4), however, they are of a limited nature and consist mainly of coordinating and organising cooperation on the most relevant immediate problems resulting mainly from difficulties in the movement of people, services and goods in connection with the pandemic and cross-border cooperation. These activities complement actions primarily at the EU level in the area of border management and strengthening cooperation among health services of its Member States.

# Index

Pages in **bold** refer tables and page followed by n refer notes.

For Product Safety Concerns and Information please contact our EU
representative GPSR@taylorandfrancis.com
Taylor & Francis Verlag GmbH, Kaufingerstraße 24, 80331 München, Germany

www.ingramcontent.com/pod-product-compliance
Lightning Source LLC
Chambersburg PA
CBHW060302220326
41598CB00027B/4202